ANTI-INFLAMMATORY PROTOCOL SANCTUARY

Rare and Delicious Recipes For Autoimmune Healing

Amelia R. Miller

COPYRIGHT

TABLE OF CONTENTS

INTRODUCTION

Welcome to this comprehensive guide to the Autoimmune Protocol (AIP) diet, a transformative approach to managing autoimmune conditions through dietary adjustments. In this book, you will embark on a journey to understand how specific foods can either contribute to inflammation or support healing and immune system regulation.

Understanding the Autoimmune Protocol

The Autoimmune Protocol (AIP) diet is designed to reduce inflammation and support immune system function by eliminating potential trigger foods and emphasizing nutrient-dense options. It goes beyond conventional dietary practices by addressing the root causes of autoimmune diseases, focusing on healing the gut, reducing inflammation, and potentially alleviating symptoms such as joint pain, fatigue, and digestive issues.

What You'll Discover

1. Comprehensive Guidance: This book provides a thorough introduction to the AIP diet, explaining its principles, benefits, and scientific basis. You'll gain insights into how specific foods impact inflammation and immune response, empowering you to make informed choices about your health.

2. Practical Advice: Expect practical tips on implementing the AIP diet in your daily life. From meal planning and grocery shopping to kitchen tips and batch cooking, you'll learn strategies to simplify the transition and maintain compliance.

3. Delicious Recipes: Explore a variety of delicious AIP-compliant recipes carefully crafted to be flavorful, satisfying, and supportive of your health goals. From nourishing breakfast options to hearty main dishes and tasty snacks, each recipe is designed to showcase the diversity and creativity possible within AIP guidelines.

4. Holistic Approach: Beyond recipes, this book explores the holistic aspects of healing, including stress management, sleep hygiene, and lifestyle practices that complement the AIP diet for comprehensive wellness.

Your Journey Starts Here

Whether you're newly diagnosed with an autoimmune condition, seeking relief from chronic symptoms, or simply exploring ways to optimize your health through diet, this book is your companion on the path to wellness. It's an invitation to take control of your health, embrace nourishing foods, and discover how simple dietary changes can have profound impacts on your well-being.

Get ready to embark on a journey of healing, empowerment, and culinary exploration with the Autoimmune Protocol diet. Your health transformation begins now.

I

Understanding the AIP Diet

The Autoimmune Protocol (AIP) diet is a specialized version of the Paleo diet designed to reduce inflammation and alleviate symptoms in individuals with autoimmune diseases. By eliminating foods that can trigger inflammation and immune responses, the AIP diet helps heal the gut and reduce the severity of autoimmune symptoms.

The AIP diet is divided into two phases: the elimination phase and the reintroduction phase. During the elimination phase, all potential inflammatory foods are removed from the diet. These include grains, legumes, dairy, eggs, nuts, seeds, nightshades (like tomatoes and peppers), processed foods, and refined sugars. Instead, the diet focuses on nutrient-dense, anti-inflammatory foods such as vegetables (excluding nightshades), fruits (in moderation), lean meats, fish, and healthy fats like avocado and coconut oil.

After the elimination phase, which typically lasts 30-90 days, the reintroduction phase begins. During this phase, foods are gradually reintroduced one at a time while monitoring for any adverse reactions. This helps identify specific food sensitivities and allows for a more personalized approach to maintaining the diet.

The AIP diet not only aims to manage symptoms but also promotes overall health by encouraging the consumption of whole, unprocessed foods rich in vitamins, minerals, and antioxidants. By supporting the body's natural healing processes, the AIP diet can be a powerful tool for individuals with autoimmune conditions.

Benefits of the AIP Diet

The Autoimmune Protocol (AIP) diet offers numerous benefits for individuals suffering from autoimmune diseases and chronic inflammation. By focusing on nutrient-dense, anti-inflammatory foods and eliminating potential dietary triggers, the AIP diet can significantly improve overall health and well-being.

One of the primary benefits of the AIP diet is its ability to reduce inflammation. Chronic inflammation is a key driver of autoimmune diseases, and by removing inflammatory foods such as grains, dairy, and processed sugars, the AIP diet helps to calm the immune system and reduce inflammation throughout the body.

Improved gut health is another significant benefit of the AIP diet. Many autoimmune conditions are linked to gut dysbiosis and leaky gut syndrome. The AIP diet promotes gut healing by eliminating foods that can damage the gut lining and introducing foods that support gut integrity and microbiome balance, such as bone broth, fermented vegetables, and high-fiber vegetables.

Additionally, the AIP diet can lead to better symptom management. Many individuals report a reduction in symptoms such as joint pain, fatigue, and digestive issues. The diet's emphasis on whole, unprocessed foods also contributes to improved nutrient intake, supporting overall health and immune function.

Finally, the AIP diet encourages a mindful approach to eating, fostering a greater awareness of food choices and their impacts on health. This can lead to more sustainable, long-term dietary habits and a healthier lifestyle overall.

How to Get Started with AIP

Embarking on the Autoimmune Protocol (AIP) diet can feel overwhelming, but with careful planning and preparation, it becomes manageable and rewarding. Here are steps to help you get started.

First, educate yourself about the AIP diet. Understanding the rationale behind food eliminations and inclusions will empower you to make informed decisions. Read books, reputable blogs, and research articles about AIP to build a solid foundation of knowledge.

Next, prepare your pantry. Remove all non-compliant foods, such as grains, dairy, legumes, nightshades, processed foods, and refined sugars. Stock up on AIP-friendly alternatives like lean meats, fish, vegetables (excluding nightshades), fruits (in moderation), healthy fats (avocado, coconut oil), and fermented foods.

Meal planning is crucial. Create a weekly meal plan and grocery list to ensure you have all the ingredients needed for AIP-compliant meals. Batch cooking and meal prepping can save time and reduce the temptation to stray from the diet.

Start gradually by integrating more AIP-friendly foods into your meals before fully committing to the elimination phase. This can make the transition smoother and less daunting.

Support is key. Join online communities, forums, or social media groups where you can share experiences, tips, and recipes with others following the AIP diet. Having a support system can provide motivation and encouragement.

Lastly, listen to your body. Pay attention to how different foods affect your symptoms and overall well-being. The AIP diet is highly individualized, so make adjustments as needed to suit your unique needs and health goals.

Personal Journey and Inspiration

My journey with the Autoimmune Protocol (AIP) diet began out of sheer necessity. Diagnosed with an autoimmune condition, I struggled with chronic pain, fatigue, and a range of debilitating symptoms that conventional treatments only partially alleviated. Desperate for relief and a better quality of life, I turned to the AIP diet as a last resort.

Initially, the idea of eliminating so many foods seemed daunting. However, as I delved into the science behind AIP, I became hopeful. I began by meticulously planning meals, educating myself on nutrient-dense foods, and embracing a whole-foods approach. The first few weeks were challenging, filled with cravings and adjustments, but the results were astonishing.

Within a month, my symptoms began to subside. The chronic pain lessened, my energy levels improved, and I felt a renewed sense of vitality. The diet not only transformed my physical health but also reshaped my relationship with food. I discovered a passion for cooking and experimenting with new recipes that adhered to AIP guidelines.

My inspiration for writing this cookbook stems from my profound personal transformation. I want to share the knowledge and recipes that have helped me reclaim my life, hoping they can offer others the same sense of healing and empowerment. This cookbook is a testament to the incredible power of food as medicine and a guide for anyone on their own journey toward better health.

Navigating the AIP Diet

Navigating the Autoimmune Protocol (AIP) diet can be challenging, especially at the beginning, but with the right strategies, it becomes manageable and rewarding. The key to successfully following the AIP diet lies in preparation, education, and a positive mindset.

Start by familiarizing yourself with the list of foods to eliminate and those that are AIP-compliant. Grains, dairy, legumes, nightshades, nuts, seeds, and processed foods are off-limits, while vegetables (excluding nightshades), fruits (in moderation), lean meats, fish, healthy fats, and fermented foods are encouraged. Keeping a comprehensive list handy can be very helpful.

Meal planning is essential. Plan your meals and snacks ahead of time to ensure you have AIP-friendly options available. Batch cooking and meal prepping can save time and prevent last-minute temptations to stray from the diet. Keep your pantry and fridge stocked with AIP staples like coconut milk, bone broth, and a variety of fresh produce.

Dining out can be tricky, but it's not impossible. Research restaurants in advance, and don't hesitate to ask questions about ingredients and food preparation. Many establishments are willing to accommodate dietary restrictions if you explain your needs clearly.

Stay connected with the AIP community through online forums, social media groups, and blogs. These platforms offer valuable support, recipe ideas, and tips from others who are also navigating the AIP journey.

Lastly, be patient with yourself. Transitioning to the AIP diet is a significant change, and it's okay to have setbacks. Focus on the positive changes in your health and well-being, and remember that every small step forward is progress.

Essential AIP Pantry Staples

Stocking your pantry with essential Autoimmune Protocol (AIP) staples is crucial for success on the diet. These staples ensure you have the ingredients needed to create nutrient-dense, anti-inflammatory meals that support your health.

Coconut Products: Coconut milk, coconut oil, and coconut flour are versatile AIP staples. Coconut milk is perfect for smoothies, soups, and curries, while coconut oil serves as a healthy cooking fat. Coconut flour is a great alternative for baking.

Vegetables: Fresh, frozen, and fermented vegetables are cornerstones of the AIP diet. Focus on a variety of non-nightshade vegetables like leafy greens, carrots, sweet potatoes, and cruciferous veggies. Fermented vegetables like sauerkraut and kimchi support gut health.

Fruits: While fruits should be consumed in moderation, having a selection of fresh and frozen fruits like berries, apples, and bananas is beneficial for snacks and desserts.

Protein Sources: Keep your pantry stocked with canned or frozen wild-caught fish, and your fridge with fresh, grass-fed meats and poultry. Bone broth is also essential for its gut-healing properties and versatility in soups and stews.

Healthy Fats: Avocado oil, extra-virgin olive oil, and lard from pasture-raised animals are excellent for cooking and adding flavor to dishes.

Herbs and Spices: While nightshade spices are off-limits, many herbs and spices like turmeric, ginger, garlic, and rosemary add flavor and anti-inflammatory benefits to your meals.

AIP-Friendly Snacks: Coconut flakes, plantain chips, and dried fruit (with no added sugar) are handy for quick, compliant snacks.

By keeping these staples on hand, you'll be well-equipped to prepare delicious and healing AIP meals.

Meal Planning and Preparation Tips

Effective meal planning and preparation are vital for success on the Autoimmune Protocol (AIP) diet. These tips can help you stay organized, save time, and ensure you always have AIP-friendly meals on hand.

1. Plan Your Weekly Menu: Take some time each week to plan your meals and snacks. Choose recipes that incorporate a variety of AIP-compliant foods to ensure balanced nutrition. Write down a detailed grocery list to avoid multiple trips to the store.

2. Batch Cooking: Prepare large quantities of staple foods, such as roasted vegetables, grilled chicken, and bone broth, to use throughout the week. Batch cooking saves time and provides ready-to-eat options, making it easier to stick to the diet.

3. Utilize Freezer-Friendly Meals: Prepare and freeze meals in advance. Soups, stews, and casseroles are excellent options for freezing. This ensures you have quick and easy meals available, especially on busy days.

4. Prep Ingredients Ahead: Wash, chop, and store vegetables in advance. Pre-cutting ingredients saves time during the week and makes meal preparation faster and more convenient.

5. Invest in Quality Storage Containers: Good storage containers keep your prepped ingredients and batch-cooked meals fresh. Glass containers are ideal as they are non-toxic and maintain the food's quality.

6. Create a Routine: Set aside specific days for meal planning, grocery shopping, and meal prepping. Establishing a routine helps streamline the process and makes it a regular part of your weekly schedule.

7. Keep Simple Recipes on Hand: Have a selection of easy, quick recipes for days when you have less time to cook. Simple stir-fries, salads, and sheet pan meals can be lifesavers.

By incorporating these tips into your routine, you'll find meal planning and preparation on the AIP diet more manageable and sustainable, ultimately supporting your journey to better health.

How to Safely Reintroduce Foods

The reintroduction phase of the Autoimmune Protocol (AIP) diet is a critical step that allows you to identify which foods trigger symptoms and which ones you can safely reintroduce into your diet. This process should be done carefully and systematically to ensure accurate results.

1. Wait for Stability: Before beginning the reintroduction phase, ensure that your symptoms have significantly improved or stabilized. This typically occurs after the initial elimination phase, which lasts between 30 to 90 days.

2. Reintroduce One Food at a Time: Introduce one new food at a time, allowing three to seven days between each reintroduction. This gap helps identify any delayed reactions and ensures that symptoms are clearly linked to the specific food being tested.

3. Start with Least Likely Offenders: Begin with foods that are less likely to cause reactions, such as egg yolks, certain seeds, and nuts.

Gradually move towards foods that are more likely to cause reactions, like dairy, grains, and nightshades.

4. Follow a Structured Method: On the first day, consume a small amount of the reintroduced food, such as a teaspoon. If no reaction occurs, increase the portion to a tablespoon on the second day, and then a larger portion on the third day. Monitor your body for any symptoms throughout this period.

5. Keep a Food Journal: Document each reintroduction, noting the food, the amount consumed, and any symptoms that arise. This journal will help track patterns and identify foods that trigger adverse reactions.

6. Be Patient and Observant: Some reactions may be subtle or delayed, so patience and keen observation are essential. If you experience symptoms, revert to the elimination phase until symptoms subside before attempting another reintroduction.

By following these guidelines, you can safely and effectively determine which foods are compatible with your body, allowing you to customize your diet for optimal health.

II

Breakfast Introduction to Anti-inflammatory Autoimmune Protocol

Starting your day with an Anti-inflammatory Autoimmune Protocol (AIP) breakfast sets a positive tone for maintaining dietary compliance and managing autoimmune symptoms. Breakfast on the AIP diet emphasizes nutrient-dense, anti-inflammatory foods that provide sustained energy and support overall health.

A typical AIP breakfast avoids common allergens like grains, dairy, and eggs, focusing instead on whole foods that nourish and heal. A nourishing AIP breakfast might include a combination of vegetables, healthy fats, and high-quality protein.

For example, a Sweet Potato and Apple Hash is a hearty and satisfying option. This dish combines roasted sweet potatoes, apples, and ground turkey, seasoned with herbs and cooked in coconut oil. The sweet potatoes provide complex carbohydrates for lasting energy, while the turkey offers lean protein, and the coconut oil supplies healthy fats.

Another excellent choice is a Banana Coconut Pancake, made from a blend of ripe bananas, coconut flour, and coconut milk. These pancakes are grain-free, dairy-free, and delicious, offering a sweet start to your day without inflammatory ingredients.

Smoothies are also a convenient and versatile breakfast option. An AIP Breakfast Smoothie might include coconut milk, frozen berries, spinach, and a scoop of collagen peptides for added protein. This nutrient-packed smoothie is easy to digest and provides a quick, nutritious meal.

By embracing creative and delicious AIP-compliant breakfast recipes, you can enjoy a variety of flavors and textures while supporting your health and well-being on the AIP diet.

Sweet Potato and Apple Hash

Ingredients:
2 medium sweet potatoes, peeled and diced

1 large apple, cored and diced (choose a variety like Granny Smith or Honeycrisp)
1/2 pound ground turkey or chicken
1 tablespoon coconut oil
1 teaspoon dried thyme
Salt and pepper to taste
Fresh parsley, chopped (optional, for garnish)

Instructions:
1. Heat coconut oil in a large skillet over medium heat.
2. Add diced sweet potatoes to the skillet and cook for about 8-10 minutes, stirring occasionally, until they begin to soften.
3. Push the sweet potatoes to one side of the skillet and add the ground turkey to the other side. Cook the turkey, breaking it apart with a spatula, until it's browned and cooked through.
4. Stir in diced apples, dried thyme, salt, and pepper. Continue cooking for another 5-7 minutes, or until the apples are tender and everything is well combined.
5. Remove from heat and garnish with chopped fresh parsley if desired.
6. Serve warm and enjoy!

Tips/Notes:
You can vary the seasoning by adding cinnamon or nutmeg for a sweeter flavor profile.
Ensure the sweet potatoes and apples are diced into similar-sized pieces for even cooking.
This dish can be made ahead and stored in the refrigerator for up to 3 days. Reheat gently on the stove or in the microwave before serving.

Nutritional Information (per serving):
Calories: 320 kcal

Protein: 20g
Carbohydrates: 35g
Fiber: 6g
Fat: 12g
Saturated Fat: 6g
Cholesterol: 50mg
Sodium: 280mg
Potassium: 800mg

This Sweet Potato and Apple Hash is a flavorful and nutrient-rich breakfast option that aligns perfectly with the Anti-inflammatory Autoimmune Protocol (AIP) diet. It provides a balance of carbohydrates, protein, and healthy fats to start your day right while supporting your health goals.

Banana Coconut Pancakes

Ingredients:
2 ripe bananas
1/4 cup coconut flour
1/4 cup coconut milk
1/2 teaspoon baking soda
1/2 teaspoon cinnamon
Coconut oil or ghee, for cooking
Fresh berries and maple syrup (optional, for serving)

Instructions:
1. In a mixing bowl, mash the ripe bananas until smooth.

2. Add coconut flour, coconut milk, baking soda, and cinnamon to the mashed bananas. Stir until well combined and a thick batter forms. If the batter seems too thick, add a little more coconut milk.
3. Heat a skillet or griddle over medium heat and lightly grease with coconut oil or ghee.
4. Spoon about 2 tablespoons of batter onto the skillet for each pancake, spreading it slightly with the back of the spoon.
5. Cook for 2-3 minutes, or until bubbles form on the surface of the pancakes and the edges look set.
6. Carefully flip the pancakes and cook for another 1-2 minutes, until golden brown and cooked through.
7. Remove from the skillet and repeat with the remaining batter.
8. Serve warm with fresh berries and a drizzle of maple syrup if desired.

Tips/Notes:
Ensure your bananas are ripe for natural sweetness and easier mashing.
Coconut flour absorbs more liquid than regular flour, so the batter should be thicker.
Adjust the cooking temperature as needed to prevent burning, as coconut flour pancakes cook slightly differently than traditional pancakes.

Nutritional Information (per serving, without toppings):
Calories: 180 kcal
Protein: 3g
Carbohydrates: 25g
Fiber: 5g
Fat: 8g
Saturated Fat: 7g
Cholesterol: 0mg
Sodium: 120mg

Potassium: 260mg

These Banana Coconut Pancakes are a delightful and nutritious option for an Anti-inflammatory Autoimmune Protocol (AIP) breakfast. They are gluten-free, dairy-free, and free of refined sugars, making them a perfect choice for anyone following an AIP diet or looking for a healthy pancake alternative.

AIP Breakfast Smoothie

Ingredients:
1 cup coconut milk (or almond milk for reintroduction phase)
1/2 cup frozen mixed berries (strawberries, blueberries, raspberries)
1/2 ripe avocado
1 tablespoon collagen peptides (optional, for added protein)
1 teaspoon fresh grated ginger
1 handful spinach leaves
Ice cubes (optional, for desired consistency)

Instructions:
1. Place all ingredients in a blender.
2. Blend on high until smooth and creamy, adjusting consistency with ice cubes if desired.
3. Pour into a glass and serve immediately.

Tips/Notes:
Use coconut milk for full AIP compliance; almond milk can be used during the reintroduction phase if tolerated.

Adjust sweetness by adding a pitted date or a teaspoon of honey (if tolerated) for a sweeter smoothie.

Fresh ginger adds a zesty kick and anti-inflammatory benefits, but adjust amount to taste.

This smoothie can be customized with other AIP-friendly ingredients like kale, cucumber, or a tablespoon of coconut oil for added fat.

Nutritional Information (per serving):
Calories: 250 kcal
Protein: 5g
Carbohydrates: 15g
Fiber: 6g
Fat: 20g
Saturated Fat: 14g
Cholesterol: 0mg
Sodium: 40mg
Potassium: 560mg

This AIP Breakfast Smoothie is packed with nutrients, antioxidants, and anti-inflammatory properties, making it an ideal choice for starting your day on the Autoimmune Protocol diet. It provides a balanced mix of protein, healthy fats, and carbohydrates to fuel your morning while supporting your health goals.

Turkey Breakfast Sausage Patties

Ingredients:
1 pound ground turkey (preferably organic)
1 teaspoon dried sage

1/2 teaspoon dried thyme
1/2 teaspoon garlic powder
1/2 teaspoon onion powder
1/4 teaspoon ground ginger
1/4 teaspoon sea salt
1/4 teaspoon black pepper (omit for strict AIP)
2 tablespoons coconut oil, for cooking

Instructions:
1. In a mixing bowl, combine ground turkey with dried sage, thyme, garlic powder, onion powder, ground ginger, sea salt, and black pepper (if using).
2. Mix well until all spices are evenly distributed throughout the turkey.
3. Divide the mixture into equal portions and shape into patties about 2-3 inches in diameter.
4. Heat coconut oil in a skillet over medium heat.
5. Cook the patties for about 4-5 minutes on each side, or until fully cooked through and golden brown.
6. Remove from the skillet and place on a paper towel-lined plate to absorb any excess oil.
7. Serve hot and enjoy!

Tips/Notes:
For strict AIP compliance, ensure spices are free from additives and fillers.
Customize the seasoning to your preference, adding more herbs or adjusting salt levels.
These patties can be made ahead of time and stored in the refrigerator for up to 3 days or frozen for longer storage. Reheat gently in a skillet or microwave before serving.

Nutritional Information (per serving, based on 4 servings):

Calories: 200 kcal
Protein: 25g
Carbohydrates: 1g
Fat: 10g
Saturated Fat: 6g
Cholesterol: 80mg
Sodium: 300mg
Potassium: 300mg

These Turkey Breakfast Sausage Patties are a flavorful and protein-packed option for an Anti-inflammatory Autoimmune Protocol (AIP) breakfast. They are free from common allergens and additives, making them suitable for those following a strict AIP diet while providing essential nutrients to start your day right.

Butternut Squash Breakfast Bowls

Ingredients:
1 small butternut squash, peeled, seeded, and cubed
1 tablespoon coconut oil
1 teaspoon cinnamon
Pinch of sea salt
1/4 cup coconut milk
1/4 cup unsweetened shredded coconut
Fresh berries or sliced banana (optional, for topping)

Instructions:
1. Preheat the oven to 400°F (200°C).
2. Toss the cubed butternut squash with coconut oil, cinnamon, and a pinch of sea salt on a baking sheet.

3. Roast in the preheated oven for 25-30 minutes, or until the squash is tender and lightly caramelized, stirring halfway through.
4. Remove from the oven and let cool slightly.
5. Transfer the roasted butternut squash to a bowl and mash with a fork or potato masher until smooth.
6. Stir in coconut milk until desired consistency is reached.
7. Divide the squash mixture into bowls and top with shredded coconut and fresh berries or sliced banana if desired.
8. Serve warm and enjoy!

Tips/Notes:
You can add a drizzle of honey or maple syrup (if tolerated) for added sweetness.
Customize your toppings with nuts, seeds, or a dollop of coconut yogurt for extra flavor and texture.
This recipe can be prepared ahead of time and stored in the refrigerator for up to 3 days. Reheat gently in the microwave or on the stove before serving.

Nutritional Information (per serving, without toppings):
Calories: 180 kcal
Protein: 2g
Carbohydrates: 20g
Fiber: 4g
Fat: 12g
Saturated Fat: 10g
Cholesterol: 0mg
Sodium: 80mg
Potassium: 480mg

This Butternut Squash Breakfast Bowl offers a comforting and nutrient-rich start to your day on the Anti-inflammatory Autoimmune Protocol (AIP) diet. It's packed with vitamins, minerals, and healthy fats, providing sustained energy and supporting overall health goals.

Carrot and Zucchini Muffins

Ingredients:
1 cup grated carrots
1 cup grated zucchini, squeezed to remove excess moisture
1/2 cup coconut flour
1/4 cup arrowroot flour
1/4 cup coconut oil, melted
3 tablespoons honey (or maple syrup for strict AIP)
3 large eggs (replace with mashed banana or applesauce for egg-free version)
1 teaspoon baking soda
1 teaspoon ground cinnamon
1/2 teaspoon ground ginger
Pinch of sea salt

Instructions:
1. Preheat the oven to 350°F (175°C) and line a muffin tin with paper liners or grease with coconut oil.
2. In a large mixing bowl, combine grated carrots, grated zucchini, coconut flour, arrowroot flour, baking soda, cinnamon, ginger, and sea salt.
3. In a separate bowl, whisk together melted coconut oil, honey (or maple syrup), and eggs (or egg substitute).
4. Pour the wet ingredients into the dry ingredients and stir until well combined.

5. Spoon the batter evenly into the prepared muffin tin, filling each cup about 3/4 full.

6. Bake for 20-25 minutes, or until the muffins are golden brown and a toothpick inserted into the center comes out clean.

7. Remove from the oven and let cool in the tin for 5 minutes before transferring to a wire rack to cool completely.

Tips/Notes:

Ensure the grated zucchini is squeezed well to remove excess moisture to prevent soggy muffins.

Add chopped nuts or seeds for added texture and crunch if tolerated.

Store leftover muffins in an airtight container in the refrigerator for up to 5 days or freeze for longer storage.

Nutritional Information (per muffin, based on 12 servings):

Calories: 120 kcal

Protein: 3g

Carbohydrates: 12g

Fiber: 3g

Fat: 7g

Saturated Fat: 5g

Cholesterol: 47mg

Sodium: 130mg

Potassium: 160mg

These Carrot and Zucchini Muffins are a delicious and nutrient-packed addition to your Anti-inflammatory Autoimmune Protocol (AIP) breakfast. They are gluten-free, dairy-free, and free from refined sugars, making them a perfect choice for a satisfying and wholesome morning treat.

AIP Granola with Coconut Yogurt

Ingredients:
1 cup unsweetened coconut flakes
1/2 cup sliced almonds
1/2 cup pumpkin seeds
1/4 cup sunflower seeds
2 tablespoons coconut oil, melted
1 tablespoon honey (or maple syrup for strict AIP)
1/2 teaspoon ground cinnamon
Pinch of sea salt
Coconut yogurt, for serving
Fresh berries or sliced fruit (optional, for serving)

Instructions:
1. Preheat the oven to 300°F (150°C) and line a baking sheet with parchment paper.
2. In a large mixing bowl, combine coconut flakes, sliced almonds, pumpkin seeds, sunflower seeds, melted coconut oil, honey (or maple syrup), ground cinnamon, and a pinch of sea salt. Mix well until all ingredients are evenly coated.
3. Spread the mixture evenly onto the prepared baking sheet.
4. Bake for 20-25 minutes, stirring halfway through, until the granola is golden brown and crispy.
5. Remove from the oven and let cool completely on the baking sheet. The granola will continue to crisp up as it cools.
6. Once cooled, transfer the granola to an airtight container for storage.
7. Serve the AIP granola with coconut yogurt and fresh berries or sliced fruit if desired.

Tips/Notes:

Ensure the granola is completely cooled before storing to maintain its crispiness.

Customize the granola by adding dried fruits like raisins or chopped apricots after baking, if tolerated.

Store leftover granola in an airtight container at room temperature for up to 2 weeks.

Nutritional Information (per serving of granola, without yogurt or toppings):

Calories: 180 kcal

Protein: 4g

Carbohydrates: 8g

Fiber: 3g

Fat: 15g

Saturated Fat: 8g

Cholesterol: 0mg

Sodium: 40mg

Potassium: 180mg

This AIP Granola with Coconut Yogurt offers a crunchy and satisfying breakfast option that adheres to the Anti-inflammatory Autoimmune Protocol (AIP) guidelines. It's rich in healthy fats, protein, and fiber, providing sustained energy and a delightful start to your day.

Berry Chia Pudding

Ingredients:
1/4 cup chia seeds
1 cup coconut milk (or almond milk for reintroduction phase)
1 tablespoon honey (or maple syrup for strict AIP)
1/2 teaspoon vanilla extract (omit for strict AIP)
1/2 cup mixed berries (fresh or frozen), plus extra for garnish
Unsweetened shredded coconut, for garnish (optional)

Instructions:
1. In a mixing bowl, combine chia seeds, coconut milk (or almond milk), honey (or maple syrup), and vanilla extract (if using). Stir well to combine.
2. Let the mixture sit for 5 minutes, then stir again to prevent clumping.
3. Cover the bowl and refrigerate for at least 2 hours, or overnight, to allow the chia seeds to absorb the liquid and thicken into a pudding-like consistency.
4. Once the chia pudding has set, stir in mixed berries.
5. Spoon the chia pudding into serving bowls or glasses.
6. Garnish with extra berries and a sprinkle of unsweetened shredded coconut if desired.
7. Serve chilled and enjoy!

Tips/Notes:
Adjust sweetness by adding more honey or maple syrup to taste. For added texture, blend half of the berries into the chia mixture before refrigerating.

Chia pudding can be stored in the refrigerator for up to 3 days. Stir well before serving, as it may thicken further.
Experiment with different types of berries or add a dash of cinnamon for extra flavor.

Nutritional Information (per serving):
Calories: 180 kcal
Protein: 4g
Carbohydrates: 17g
Fiber: 8g
Fat: 12g
Saturated Fat: 7g
Cholesterol: 0mg
Sodium: 20mg
Potassium: 220mg

This Berry Chia Pudding is a nutritious and satisfying option for an Anti-inflammatory Autoimmune Protocol (AIP) breakfast. It's packed with fiber, antioxidants from berries, and healthy fats from chia seeds and coconut milk, making it an excellent choice for supporting your health and well-being.

Plantain and Avocado Toast

Ingredients:
1 ripe plantain, peeled and sliced
1 tablespoon coconut oil
1 ripe avocado
Juice of 1/2 lime
Pinch of sea salt

Pinch of red pepper flakes (optional)
Fresh cilantro leaves, chopped (optional, for garnish)
Sliced cucumber or radish (optional, for topping)

Instructions:
1. Heat coconut oil in a skillet over medium heat.
2. Add sliced plantain to the skillet and cook for 2-3 minutes per side, or until golden brown and caramelized.
3. While the plantains are cooking, mash the ripe avocado in a bowl with lime juice, sea salt, and red pepper flakes (if using).
4. Toast your favorite AIP-compliant bread or bread alternative until golden brown and crispy.
5. Spread the mashed avocado mixture evenly onto the toasted bread slices.
6. Top each slice with cooked plantain slices.
7. Garnish with fresh cilantro leaves and sliced cucumber or radish if desired.
8. Serve immediately and enjoy!

Tips/Notes:
Choose a ripe plantain that is yellow with some black spots for sweetness.
Adjust the amount of lime juice and sea salt to taste for the avocado mash.
Plantain slices can also be grilled for a smokier flavor.
This toast is delicious with additional toppings like sliced tomatoes or a sprinkle of nutritional yeast.

Nutritional Information (per serving, based on 2 servings):
Calories: 280 kcal
Protein: 3g
Carbohydrates: 30g
Fiber: 6g

Fat: 18g
Saturated Fat: 10g
Cholesterol: 0mg
Sodium: 150mg
Potassium: 810mg

This Plantain and Avocado Toast is a unique and flavorful breakfast option that adheres to the Anti-inflammatory Autoimmune Protocol (AIP) guidelines. It combines the sweetness of caramelized plantains with creamy avocado and tangy lime, creating a satisfying and nutrient-dense meal to start your day right.

Pumpkin Spice Smoothie

Ingredients:
1/2 cup canned pumpkin puree (unsweetened)
1/2 cup coconut milk
1 ripe banana
1 tablespoon almond butter (or sunflower seed butter for nut-free)
1 tablespoon maple syrup (or honey for strict AIP)
1/2 teaspoon ground cinnamon
1/4 teaspoon ground ginger
1/8 teaspoon ground nutmeg
1/8 teaspoon ground cloves
Ice cubes (optional, for desired consistency)

Instructions:
1. Place all ingredients in a blender.

2. Blend on high until smooth and creamy, adjusting consistency with ice cubes if desired.
3. Pour into a glass and sprinkle with additional cinnamon or nutmeg for garnish if desired.
4. Serve immediately and enjoy!

Tips/Notes:
Use canned pumpkin puree without added sugar or spices for full AIP compliance.
Adjust sweetness by adding more or less maple syrup or honey according to your taste preference.
For a thicker smoothie, freeze the banana slices before blending.
This smoothie can be made ahead and stored in the refrigerator for up to 24 hours. Stir well before serving.

Nutritional Information (per serving):
Calories: 250 kcal
Protein: 4g
Carbohydrates: 30g
Fiber: 5g
Fat: 14g
Saturated Fat: 8g
Cholesterol: 0mg
Sodium: 30mg
Potassium: 540mg

This Pumpkin Spice Smoothie is a delicious and seasonal treat that aligns perfectly with the Anti-inflammatory Autoimmune Protocol (AIP) guidelines. It's rich in fiber, vitamins, and minerals from pumpkin and spices, providing a comforting and nutritious option for your morning routine.

Cauliflower Breakfast Fried Rice

Ingredients:
1 small head cauliflower, grated or processed into rice-like consistency
1 tablespoon coconut oil
2 cloves garlic, minced
1/2 onion, finely chopped
1/2 red bell pepper, diced
1/2 cup diced cooked chicken or turkey (optional)
2 tablespoons coconut aminos
1 teaspoon ground ginger
1/2 teaspoon sea salt
2 green onions, sliced (optional, for garnish)
Fresh cilantro leaves, chopped (optional, for garnish)

Instructions:
1. Heat coconut oil in a large skillet or wok over medium-high heat.
2. Add minced garlic and chopped onion to the skillet. Saute for 2-3 minutes until fragrant and onions are translucent.
3. Add diced red bell pepper and cook for another 2 minutes, stirring occasionally.
4. Push the vegetables to one side of the skillet and add grated cauliflower. Cook for 5-6 minutes, stirring frequently, until cauliflower is tender and slightly golden.
5. Stir in diced cooked chicken or turkey (if using), coconut aminos, ground ginger, and sea salt. Cook for another 2-3 minutes until heated through and well combined.
6. Remove from heat and garnish with sliced green onions and chopped cilantro if desired.

7. Serve hot and enjoy!

Tips/Notes:
Ensure the cauliflower rice is dried well after grating or processing to avoid excess moisture in the fried rice.
Customize with additional vegetables like peas, carrots, or broccoli for added nutrition and color.
Use tamari or soy sauce (if tolerated) instead of coconut aminos for a different flavor profile.
This cauliflower fried rice can be stored in an airtight container in the refrigerator for up to 3 days. Reheat gently in a skillet or microwave before serving.

Nutritional Information (per serving, based on 4 servings):
Calories: 120 kcal
Protein: 8g
Carbohydrates: 10g
Fiber: 4g
Fat: 6g
Saturated Fat: 4g
Cholesterol: 15mg
Sodium: 300mg
Potassium: 520mg

This Cauliflower Breakfast Fried Rice is a flavorful and nutrient-packed option for an Anti-inflammatory Autoimmune Protocol (AIP) breakfast. It's low in carbohydrates, gluten-free, and dairy-free, making it suitable for those following an AIP diet while providing essential nutrients to start your day right.

Apple Cinnamon Breakfast Bars

Ingredients:
2 cups shredded apples (about 2 medium apples, peeled and cored)
1 cup coconut flour
1/2 cup shredded coconut (unsweetened)
1/2 cup raisins or chopped dried apples (unsweetened)
1/4 cup coconut oil, melted
1/4 cup maple syrup (or honey for strict AIP)
2 teaspoons ground cinnamon
1/2 teaspoon ground ginger
Pinch of sea salt

Instructions:
1. Preheat the oven to 350°F (175°C) and line a baking dish with parchment paper.
2. In a large mixing bowl, combine shredded apples, coconut flour, shredded coconut, raisins or chopped dried apples, melted coconut oil, maple syrup (or honey), ground cinnamon, ground ginger, and a pinch of sea salt. Mix well until all ingredients are evenly combined and a thick batter forms.
3. Press the mixture firmly and evenly into the prepared baking dish.
4. Bake for 25-30 minutes, or until the bars are golden brown and firm to the touch.
5. Remove from the oven and let cool completely in the baking dish before cutting into bars or squares.
6. Once cooled, store in an airtight container at room temperature or in the refrigerator for up to 5 days.

Tips/Notes:

Use a box grater or food processor to shred the apples.

Adjust sweetness by adding more or less maple syrup or honey according to your taste preference.

For added crunch, sprinkle chopped nuts or seeds on top of the batter before baking.

These breakfast bars are perfect for meal prep and can be enjoyed on the go or as a quick breakfast option.

Nutritional Information (per serving, based on 12 servings):
Calories: 150 kcal
Protein: 2g
Carbohydrates: 20g
Fiber: 4g
Fat: 8g
Saturated Fat: 6g
Cholesterol: 0mg
Sodium: 40mg
Potassium: 160mg

These Apple Cinnamon Breakfast Bars are a wholesome and satisfying choice for an Anti-inflammatory Autoimmune Protocol (AIP) breakfast. They are gluten-free, dairy-free, and free from refined sugars, making them a nutritious option to fuel your day while adhering to your dietary preferences.

III

Snacks and Treats

Incorporating snacks and treats into an Anti-inflammatory Autoimmune Protocol (AIP) can be both enjoyable and supportive of your health goals. Snacks and treats on the AIP focus on nutrient-dense ingredients that avoid common inflammatory triggers such as gluten, dairy, processed sugars, and additives.

AIP snacks often feature whole foods like fruits, vegetables, nuts (if tolerated), seeds, and healthy fats like coconut oil or avocado. These snacks not only provide sustenance between meals but also contribute essential vitamins, minerals, and antioxidants that support overall well-being.

Treats within the AIP framework are typically made using AIP-compliant ingredients such as coconut flour, cassava flour, and natural sweeteners like honey or maple syrup (in moderation). These treats can include baked goods like muffins, cookies, or bars that are free from grains, dairy, and refined sugars, yet still satisfy cravings for something sweet.

By focusing on nutrient density and avoiding inflammatory ingredients, snacks and treats on the AIP promote gut health, reduce inflammation, and support immune function. They offer a variety of flavors and textures that make adhering to the AIP more sustainable and enjoyable, allowing individuals to explore delicious alternatives while maintaining a balanced approach to their dietary needs.

Crispy Kale Chips

Ingredients:
1 bunch kale (about 8-10 large leaves)
1 tablespoon olive oil
Sea salt, to taste

Instructions:
1. Preheat the oven to 275°F (135°C) and line a baking sheet with parchment paper.
2. Wash the kale leaves thoroughly and pat them dry with a paper towel or kitchen towel.
3. Remove the tough stems from the kale leaves and tear the leaves into bite-sized pieces.
4. In a large mixing bowl, drizzle olive oil over the kale leaves and massage the oil into the leaves until they are evenly coated.
5. Arrange the kale pieces in a single layer on the prepared baking sheet.
6. Sprinkle sea salt lightly over the kale chips.
7. Bake in the preheated oven for 20-25 minutes, or until the kale chips are crispy and slightly golden, checking and turning halfway through baking.

8. Remove from the oven and let cool on the baking sheet for a few minutes before transferring to a wire rack to cool completely.

Tips/Notes:
Ensure the kale leaves are thoroughly dried after washing to achieve crispy chips.
Experiment with different seasonings such as garlic powder, onion powder, or nutritional yeast for added flavor.
Kale chips can burn easily, so keep an eye on them during the last few minutes of baking.
Store leftover kale chips in an airtight container at room temperature for up to 3 days for optimal crispiness.

Nutritional Information (per serving, based on 2 servings):
Calories: 80 kcal
Protein: 3g
Carbohydrates: 6g
Fiber: 1g
Fat: 5g
Saturated Fat: 1g
Cholesterol: 0mg
Sodium: 150mg
Potassium: 350mg

Crispy Kale Chips are a nutritious and crunchy snack option that aligns with the Anti-inflammatory Autoimmune Protocol (AIP) guidelines. They are rich in vitamins, minerals, and antioxidants while being low in calories and carbohydrates, making them an excellent choice for satisfying cravings while supporting your health goals.

Baked Plantain Chips

Ingredients:
2 ripe plantains
2 tablespoons coconut oil, melted
Sea salt, to taste

Instructions:
1. Preheat the oven to 400°F (200°C) and line a baking sheet with parchment paper.
2. Peel the plantains and thinly slice them into rounds using a sharp knife or mandoline slicer.
3. Place the plantain slices in a mixing bowl and toss with melted coconut oil until evenly coated.
4. Arrange the plantain slices in a single layer on the prepared baking sheet.
5. Sprinkle sea salt lightly over the plantain slices.
6. Bake in the preheated oven for 15-20 minutes, flipping the slices halfway through, until the plantain chips are golden brown and crispy.
7. Remove from the oven and let cool on the baking sheet for a few minutes before transferring to a wire rack to cool completely.

Tips/Notes:
Use ripe plantains that are yellow with some black spots for sweetness.
Adjust the thickness of the slices for varying textures of chips.
For extra flavor, sprinkle with additional seasonings such as cinnamon or paprika before baking.

Store leftover plantain chips in an airtight container at room temperature for up to 3 days for optimal crispiness.

Nutritional Information (per serving, based on 2 servings):
Calories: 180 kcal
Protein: 1g
Carbohydrates: 30g
Fiber: 2g
Fat: 8g
Saturated Fat: 7g
Cholesterol: 0mg
Sodium: 150mg
Potassium: 450mg

Baked Plantain Chips are a crunchy and satisfying snack option that fits well within the Anti-inflammatory Autoimmune Protocol (AIP) guidelines. They are free from grains, gluten, and refined sugars, making them a nutritious alternative to traditional chips while providing essential vitamins and minerals from plantains and coconut oil.

AIP Guacamole with Veggie Sticks

Ingredients:
2 ripe avocados
1/4 cup finely chopped red onion
1/4 cup chopped fresh cilantro
Juice of 1 lime
1/2 teaspoon sea salt
1/4 teaspoon ground cumin (omit for strict AIP)

Carrot sticks, cucumber sticks, and bell pepper strips, for serving

Instructions:
1. Cut the avocados in half, remove the pits, and scoop the flesh into a mixing bowl.
2. Mash the avocados with a fork until smooth or chunky, depending on your preference.
3. Add chopped red onion, chopped cilantro, lime juice, sea salt, and ground cumin (if using).
4. Stir well to combine all ingredients thoroughly.
5. Taste and adjust seasoning if needed, adding more lime juice or sea salt as desired.
6. Serve the guacamole immediately with carrot sticks, cucumber sticks, and bell pepper strips for dipping.

Tips/Notes:
For a smoother guacamole, use a food processor or blender to combine the ingredients.
Keep the avocado pits in the guacamole until serving to help prevent browning.
Customize your guacamole with additional ingredients such as diced tomatoes or minced garlic, if tolerated.
Store leftover guacamole in an airtight container in the refrigerator. Press plastic wrap directly onto the surface of the guacamole to minimize exposure to air and prevent browning.

Nutritional Information (per serving, based on 4 servings):
Calories: 150 kcal
Protein: 2g
Carbohydrates: 10g
Fiber: 7g
Fat: 13g
Saturated Fat: 2g

Cholesterol: 0mg
Sodium: 300mg
Potassium: 570mg

This AIP Guacamole with Veggie Sticks is a delicious and nutrient-dense snack option that adheres to the Anti-inflammatory Autoimmune Protocol (AIP) guidelines. It's rich in healthy fats from avocados and provides essential vitamins and minerals, while the fresh vegetables offer crunch and additional nutrients. Enjoy this flavorful dip as a satisfying and nourishing addition to your AIP snacks.

Coconut Date Energy Balls

Ingredients:
1 cup pitted dates
1/2 cup shredded coconut (unsweetened), plus extra for coating
1/2 cup raw cashews
1 tablespoon coconut oil, melted
1 tablespoon water (as needed)
Pinch of sea salt

Instructions:
1. Place pitted dates, shredded coconut, raw cashews, melted coconut oil, and a pinch of sea salt in a food processor.
2. Pulse until the ingredients are finely chopped and start to come together into a sticky dough-like consistency.
3. If the mixture seems dry, add water, 1 teaspoon at a time, until the mixture sticks together easily when pressed between your fingers.

4. Scoop out tablespoon-sized portions of the mixture and roll into balls using your hands.
5. Roll each ball in additional shredded coconut to coat evenly.
6. Place the coconut date energy balls on a plate or baking sheet lined with parchment paper.
7. Refrigerate for at least 30 minutes to allow the balls to firm up.
8. Store in an airtight container in the refrigerator for up to 2 weeks.

Tips/Notes:
Use soft, moist dates for easier blending and smoother texture.
Customize the energy balls by adding cocoa powder, vanilla extract, or spices like cinnamon or nutmeg for additional flavor.
If you prefer a nut-free version, replace the cashews with sunflower seeds or pumpkin seeds.
These energy balls are perfect for a quick snack or on-the-go energy boost, packed with natural sweetness and healthy fats.

Nutritional Information (per serving, based on 12 servings):
Calories: 110 kcal
Protein: 2g
Carbohydrates: 15g
Fiber: 2g
Fat: 6g
Saturated Fat: 3g
Cholesterol: 0mg
Sodium: 10mg
Potassium: 180mg

These Coconut Date Energy Balls are a delicious and nutritious snack option that aligns with the Anti-inflammatory Autoimmune Protocol (AIP) guidelines. They provide a natural source of energy from dates and nuts, with the added benefits of fiber and healthy fats from coconut and cashews. Enjoy these bite-sized treats as a guilt-free indulgence that supports your dietary preferences and health goals.

Sweet Potato Fries

Ingredients:
2 large sweet potatoes
2 tablespoons olive oil or avocado oil
1 teaspoon garlic powder
1 teaspoon paprika
1/2 teaspoon sea salt
Freshly ground black pepper, to taste

Instructions:
1. Preheat the oven to 425°F (220°C) and line a baking sheet with parchment paper.
2. Wash and peel the sweet potatoes, then cut them into evenly sized fries or wedges.
3. In a large mixing bowl, toss sweet potato fries with olive oil or avocado oil until well coated.
4. Sprinkle garlic powder, paprika, sea salt, and freshly ground black pepper over the fries. Toss again to evenly distribute the seasonings.
5. Arrange the sweet potato fries in a single layer on the prepared baking sheet, ensuring they are not overcrowded.
6. Bake in the preheated oven for 25-30 minutes, flipping halfway through, until the fries are crispy and golden brown.
7. Remove from the oven and let cool slightly before serving.

Tips/Notes:

For crispier fries, spread them out with space between each fry on the baking sheet.

Experiment with different seasonings such as chili powder, cumin, or rosemary for added flavor variations.

Serve sweet potato fries with AIP-compliant dips like guacamole or a coconut yogurt-based dip.

Leftover sweet potato fries can be stored in an airtight container in the refrigerator for up to 3 days. Reheat in the oven or toaster oven for best results.

Nutritional Information (per serving, based on 4 servings):

Calories: 180 kcal

Protein: 2g

Carbohydrates: 26g

Fiber: 4g

Fat: 8g

Saturated Fat: 1g

Cholesterol: 0mg

Sodium: 320mg

Potassium: 470mg

These Sweet Potato Fries are a tasty and satisfying side dish or snack option that fits within the Anti-inflammatory Autoimmune Protocol (AIP) guidelines. They are rich in vitamins, minerals, and fiber from sweet potatoes, offering a nutritious alternative to traditional fries while supporting your health and dietary needs.

Carob Coconut Fudge

Ingredients:
1 cup coconut butter
1/4 cup coconut oil, melted
1/4 cup carob powder
3 tablespoons maple syrup (or honey for strict AIP)
1 teaspoon vanilla extract (omit for strict AIP)
Pinch of sea salt
Unsweetened shredded coconut, for garnish (optional)

Instructions:
1. Line a square baking dish or container with parchment paper, leaving some overhang for easy removal.
2. In a microwave-safe bowl or on the stovetop, melt coconut butter and coconut oil until smooth and liquid.
3. Stir in carob powder, maple syrup (or honey), vanilla extract (if using), and a pinch of sea salt until well combined and smooth.
4. Pour the mixture into the prepared baking dish, spreading it out evenly with a spatula.
5. Sprinkle unsweetened shredded coconut on top for garnish, if desired.
6. Refrigerate for at least 1 hour, or until the fudge is firm and set.
7. Once firm, lift the fudge out of the dish using the parchment paper overhang and cut into small squares or bars.

Tips/Notes:
Coconut butter can be found in health food stores or made by blending shredded coconut until smooth.

Adjust sweetness by adding more or less maple syrup or honey according to your taste preference.

Store leftover fudge in an airtight container in the refrigerator for up to 2 weeks or in the freezer for longer storage.

Enjoy this carob coconut fudge as a decadent treat that satisfies cravings while adhering to the Anti-inflammatory Autoimmune Protocol (AIP) guidelines.

Nutritional Information (per serving, based on 12 servings):
Calories: 180 kcal
Protein: 1g
Carbohydrates: 10g
Fiber: 2g
Fat: 16g
Saturated Fat: 13g
Cholesterol: 0mg
Sodium: 5mg
Potassium: 110mg

This Carob Coconut Fudge offers a deliciously creamy and satisfying treat that meets the criteria of the Anti-inflammatory Autoimmune Protocol (AIP). It's free from dairy, gluten, and refined sugars, making it a guilt-free indulgence packed with healthy fats from coconut butter and coconut oil.

Dehydrated Apple Slices

Ingredients:
4-5 medium apples (use sweet varieties like Gala or Fuji)
Lemon juice (optional, to prevent browning)

Instructions:
1. Wash the apples thoroughly under cold water.
2. Core the apples and slice them thinly, about 1/8 inch thick. A mandoline slicer can be helpful for achieving uniform slices.
3. Optional: To prevent browning, you can dip the apple slices in lemon juice diluted with water (1 tablespoon lemon juice to 1 cup water) for a few seconds.
4. Arrange the apple slices in a single layer on dehydrator trays, ensuring they do not overlap.
5. Set the dehydrator temperature to 135°F (57°C) and dehydrate the apple slices for 6-8 hours, or until they are dried and leathery but still pliable.
6. Rotate the trays halfway through the drying process to ensure even drying.
7. Once dried, let the apple slices cool completely before storing.

Tips/Notes:
Adjust the drying time depending on the thickness of your apple slices and your dehydrator model.
Store dehydrated apple slices in an airtight container or resealable bags in a cool, dry place. They can also be stored in the refrigerator or freezer for longer shelf life.
Enjoy dehydrated apple slices as a nutritious snack on their own or use them in trail mixes, granola, or as a topping for oatmeal and yogurt.

Nutritional Information (per serving, based on 1 medium apple):
Calories: 95 kcal
Protein: 0.5g
Carbohydrates: 25g
Fiber: 4g
Fat: 0.3g

Saturated Fat: 0.1g
Cholesterol: 0mg
Sodium: 1mg
Potassium: 195mg

Dehydrated apple slices are a wholesome snack option that retains the natural sweetness and nutrients of fresh apples. They are rich in fiber and vitamins, making them a perfect choice for those following the Anti-inflammatory Autoimmune Protocol (AIP) looking for convenient and nutritious snacks.

AIP Trail Mix

Ingredients:
1 cup coconut flakes (unsweetened)
1 cup dried apple slices, chopped
1 cup dried mango slices, chopped
1/2 cup pumpkin seeds (pepitas)
1/2 cup sunflower seeds
1/2 cup coconut chips or shreds (unsweetened)
1/2 cup dried cranberries (sweetened with apple juice or omit for strict AIP)

Instructions:
1. In a large mixing bowl, combine all the ingredients: coconut flakes, chopped dried apple slices, chopped dried mango slices, pumpkin seeds, sunflower seeds, coconut chips or shreds, and dried cranberries (if using).
2. Toss the ingredients together until evenly mixed.

3. Store the AIP trail mix in an airtight container or portion into resealable bags for convenient snacking.

Tips/Notes:

Customize your trail mix by adding other AIP-friendly dried fruits such as pineapple, apricots, or raisins.

For added crunch, include AIP-compliant nuts like chopped almonds or walnuts (if tolerated).

If avoiding dried cranberries due to added sugars, substitute with additional dried fruits or omit altogether.

Enjoy this AIP trail mix as a portable snack or energy booster during outdoor activities, hikes, or as a quick snack between meals.

Nutritional Information (per serving, based on 1/4 cup serving):

Calories: 180 kcal

Protein: 3g

Carbohydrates: 22g

Fiber: 4g

Fat: 10g

Saturated Fat: 5g

Cholesterol: 0mg

Sodium: 5mg

Potassium: 240mg

This AIP Trail Mix offers a balanced blend of flavors and textures while adhering to the Anti-inflammatory Autoimmune Protocol (AIP) guidelines. It provides a mix of healthy fats, fiber, and natural sweetness from dried fruits, making it a satisfying and nutrient-dense snack option for those with dietary restrictions or preferences.

Roasted Beet Chips

Ingredients:
3-4 medium beets, peeled and thinly sliced (about 1/16 inch thick)
2 tablespoons olive oil or avocado oil
Sea salt, to taste
Freshly ground black pepper, to taste (omit for strict AIP)

Instructions:
1. Preheat the oven to 350°F (175°C) and line a baking sheet with parchment paper.
2. Peel the beets and thinly slice them into rounds using a sharp knife or mandoline slicer.
3. In a large mixing bowl, toss beet slices with olive oil or avocado oil until well coated.
4. Arrange the beet slices in a single layer on the prepared baking sheet, ensuring they do not overlap.
5. Sprinkle sea salt and freshly ground black pepper (if using) lightly over the beet slices.
6. Bake in the preheated oven for 20-25 minutes, flipping the slices halfway through, until the beet chips are crispy and slightly curled at the edges.
7. Remove from the oven and let cool on the baking sheet for a few minutes before transferring to a wire rack to cool completely.

Tips/Notes:
Use gloves when handling beets to avoid staining your hands.
Adjust the thickness of the beet slices for varying textures of chips.
Experiment with different seasonings such as garlic powder, rosemary, or thyme for added flavor variations.

Store leftover beet chips in an airtight container at room temperature for up to 3 days for optimal crispiness.

Nutritional Information (per serving, based on 4 servings):
Calories: 90 kcal
Protein: 2g
Carbohydrates: 10g
Fiber: 3g
Fat: 5g
Saturated Fat: 1g
Cholesterol: 0mg
Sodium: 150mg
Potassium: 320mg

These Roasted Beet Chips are a colorful and crunchy snack option that aligns with the Anti-inflammatory Autoimmune Protocol (AIP) guidelines. They are packed with vitamins, minerals, and antioxidants from beets, offering a nutritious alternative to traditional chips while supporting your health and dietary needs.

AIP Popcorn (Popped Sorghum)

Ingredients:
1/2 cup whole sorghum grain
1 tablespoon coconut oil or avocado oil
Sea salt, to taste

Instructions:
1. Rinse the sorghum grain under cold water in a fine-mesh sieve.

2. In a large, heavy-bottomed pot with a lid, heat coconut oil or avocado oil over medium-high heat.

3. Add a few sorghum grains to the pot and cover with the lid slightly ajar. Wait until the grains start popping.

4. Once popping begins, quickly add the remaining sorghum grains and cover the pot completely with the lid.

5. Shake the pot gently back and forth over the heat to prevent burning and ensure even popping.

6. Continue to shake the pot until the popping slows down, about 2-3 minutes.

7. Remove from heat immediately once most of the grains have popped. Be cautious as sorghum can burn quickly.

8. Transfer the popped sorghum to a large bowl and season with sea salt to taste.

Tips/Notes:

Sorghum grains are smaller than traditional popcorn kernels and will pop into tiny, crunchy pieces.

Be careful not to overcrowd the pot, as this can prevent even popping.

Experiment with different seasonings such as nutritional yeast, garlic powder, or smoked paprika for flavor variations.

Popped sorghum can be stored in an airtight container at room temperature for up to a week.

Nutritional Information (per serving, based on 1/2 cup popped sorghum):

Calories: 100 kcal

Protein: 3g

Carbohydrates: 22g

Fiber: 3g

Fat: 1g

Saturated Fat: 0g

Cholesterol: 0mg
Sodium: 0mg
Potassium: 110mg

AIP Popcorn made from popped sorghum is a crunchy and nutritious snack option that aligns with the Anti-inflammatory Autoimmune Protocol (AIP) guidelines. It's gluten-free, grain-free, and free from common allergens, providing a satisfying alternative to traditional popcorn while offering essential nutrients and fiber from sorghum. Enjoy this light and flavorful snack for a guilt-free treat that supports your dietary preferences and health goals.

Honey-Lime Jicama Sticks

Ingredients:
1 medium jicama, peeled and cut into sticks
Juice of 1 lime
1 tablespoon honey (omit for strict AIP)
Pinch of sea salt
Fresh cilantro leaves, chopped (optional, for garnish)

Instructions:
1. Peel the jicama using a vegetable peeler and cut it into sticks resembling French fries or matchsticks.
2. In a large mixing bowl, combine jicama sticks with lime juice, honey (if using), and a pinch of sea salt. Toss well to coat evenly.
3. Transfer the jicama sticks to a serving plate or bowl.
4. Garnish with chopped fresh cilantro leaves, if desired.

5. Serve immediately as a refreshing and crunchy snack or appetizer.

Tips/Notes:
Jicama has a mild, slightly sweet flavor and a crunchy texture, making it perfect for raw snacks.
Adjust the amount of lime juice and honey according to your taste preference.
For a variation, sprinkle with chili powder or paprika for a hint of spice.
Store any leftover jicama sticks in an airtight container in the refrigerator for up to 2 days.

Nutritional Information (per serving, based on 1 medium jicama):
Calories: 50 kcal
Protein: 1g
Carbohydrates: 12g
Fiber: 6g
Fat: 0g
Saturated Fat: 0g
Cholesterol: 0mg
Sodium: 5mg
Potassium: 280mg

Honey-Lime Jicama Sticks are a refreshing and nutritious snack option that aligns with the Anti-inflammatory Autoimmune Protocol (AIP) guidelines. They are low in calories and fat, high in fiber and vitamin C, and offer a satisfying crunch. Enjoy these jicama sticks as a light and flavorful alternative to traditional snacks, perfect for serving at parties or enjoying on a sunny day.

Frozen Mango Coconut Bites

Ingredients:
1 cup frozen mango chunks
1/2 cup coconut cream
2 tablespoons shredded coconut (unsweetened)
1 tablespoon maple syrup (optional, omit for strict AIP)
1/2 teaspoon vanilla extract (omit for strict AIP)
Pinch of sea salt

Instructions:
1. In a blender or food processor, combine frozen mango chunks, coconut cream, shredded coconut, maple syrup (if using), vanilla extract (if using), and a pinch of sea salt.
2. Blend until smooth and creamy, scraping down the sides as needed to ensure all ingredients are well combined.
3. Spoon the mixture into silicone molds or ice cube trays, filling each mold or cube about three-quarters full.
4. Tap the molds or trays gently on the countertop to remove any air bubbles and smooth the tops.
5. Insert a toothpick or small skewer into each mold or cube to create a handle for easier handling.
6. Freeze the mango coconut bites for at least 4 hours, or until firm and set.
7. Once frozen, remove the bites from the molds or trays and transfer them to a freezer-safe container or resealable bag for storage.

Tips/Notes:
Use ripe and sweet mango for the best flavor.

If you prefer a sweeter treat, adjust the amount of maple syrup or substitute with honey (if tolerated).

Customize your frozen mango coconut bites by adding a sprinkle of cinnamon, nutmeg, or lime zest for additional flavor.

Enjoy these frozen treats straight from the freezer as a refreshing and creamy dessert or snack.

Nutritional Information (per bite, based on 12 servings):
Calories: 50 kcal
Protein: 0.5g
Carbohydrates: 6g
Fiber: 1g
Fat: 3g
Saturated Fat: 2.5g
Cholesterol: 0mg
Sodium: 5mg
Potassium: 60mg

These Frozen Mango Coconut Bites are a delightful and creamy dessert option that adheres to the Anti-inflammatory Autoimmune Protocol (AIP) guidelines. They are dairy-free, gluten-free, and free from refined sugars, making them a guilt-free indulgence packed with natural sweetness from mango and coconut. Enjoy these bites as a cool and satisfying treat on warm days or anytime you crave a tropical-flavored snack.

IV

Vegetarian and Vegan

Adapting the Anti-inflammatory Autoimmune Protocol (AIP) to accommodate vegetarian and vegan diets involves careful planning to ensure nutritional adequacy while adhering to the protocol's principles of reducing inflammation and supporting immune health. For vegetarians, who may include dairy and eggs in their diet, options like grass-fed ghee or clarified butter, and organic eggs can provide essential nutrients while avoiding inflammatory triggers. However, strict adherence to AIP excludes these items, focusing instead on nutrient-dense plant foods and sustainable protein sources.

Vegans following AIP omit all animal products, relying on a variety of plant-based foods such as fruits, vegetables, nuts, seeds, and gluten-free grains like quinoa or millet. To meet protein needs, legumes and beans are typically avoided during the elimination phase due to their potential inflammatory properties. Instead, sources like chia seeds, hemp seeds, and tofu can be utilized cautiously after the reintroduction phase.

Both vegetarian and vegan adaptations of AIP emphasize nutrient-rich whole foods and emphasize anti-inflammatory ingredients like turmeric, ginger, and leafy greens. Careful meal planning is essential to ensure adequate intake of vitamins, minerals, and essential fatty acids, potentially supplementing with vitamins B12 and D if needed. With thoughtful planning and creativity, vegetarian and vegan versions of AIP can provide a balanced approach to managing autoimmune conditions while promoting overall health and wellness.

Roasted Vegetable Medley

Ingredients:
2 cups Brussels sprouts, trimmed and halved
1 large sweet potato, peeled and cut into cubes
1 red bell pepper, seeded and chopped
1 yellow bell pepper, seeded and chopped
1 medium red onion, sliced
2 tablespoons olive oil or avocado oil
1 teaspoon dried thyme
1 teaspoon dried rosemary
Sea salt and freshly ground black pepper, to taste

Instructions:
1. Preheat the oven to 400°F (200°C) and line a baking sheet with parchment paper.
2. In a large mixing bowl, combine Brussels sprouts, sweet potato cubes, chopped red bell pepper, chopped yellow bell pepper, and sliced red onion.

3. Drizzle olive oil or avocado oil over the vegetables and toss to coat evenly.

4. Sprinkle dried thyme, dried rosemary, sea salt, and freshly ground black pepper over the vegetables. Toss again to distribute the seasonings.

5. Spread the vegetable mixture in a single layer on the prepared baking sheet.

6. Roast in the preheated oven for 25-30 minutes, stirring halfway through, until the vegetables are tender and caramelized.

7. Remove from the oven and let cool slightly before serving.

Tips/Notes:

Cut the vegetables into similar-sized pieces for even cooking.

Add garlic cloves or shallots for extra flavor, if desired.

Serve the roasted vegetable medley as a side dish or main course with protein of choice, such as grilled chicken or tofu.

Leftovers can be stored in an airtight container in the refrigerator for up to 3 days.

Nutritional Information (per serving, based on 4 servings):

Calories: 180 kcal

Protein: 3g

Carbohydrates: 25g

Fiber: 6g

Fat: 8g

Saturated Fat: 1g

Cholesterol: 0mg

Sodium: 60mg

Potassium: 680mg

This Roasted Vegetable Medley is a colorful and nutritious dish that aligns with the principles of the Anti-inflammatory Autoimmune Protocol (AIP). It's rich in fiber, vitamins, and antioxidants from a variety of vegetables, offering a satisfying and flavorful addition to any meal. Enjoy the natural sweetness and earthy flavors of roasted Brussels sprouts, sweet potatoes, and bell peppers, enhanced with aromatic herbs for a wholesome and comforting dish that supports your health and wellness goals.

Cauliflower "Rice" Stir Fry

Ingredients:
1 head cauliflower, grated or processed into rice-like grains
1 tablespoon coconut oil or avocado oil
1 onion, finely chopped
2 cloves garlic, minced
1 carrot, diced
1 red bell pepper, diced
1 cup broccoli florets
1/2 cup snow peas, trimmed
2 tablespoons coconut aminos (or tamari sauce for non-AIP)
1 teaspoon grated ginger
Sea salt and freshly ground black pepper, to taste
Fresh cilantro, chopped (optional, for garnish)

Instructions:
1. Grate or process the cauliflower into rice-sized pieces using a food processor or box grater.
2. Heat coconut oil or avocado oil in a large skillet or wok over medium heat.
3. Add chopped onion and minced garlic to the skillet, sautéing until fragrant and translucent.

4. Stir in diced carrot, diced red bell pepper, broccoli florets, and snow peas, cooking until vegetables are tender-crisp.

5. Add cauliflower rice to the skillet, stirring well to combine with the vegetables.

6. Drizzle coconut aminos (or tamari sauce), grated ginger, sea salt, and freshly ground black pepper over the cauliflower rice mixture. Stir-fry for 5-7 minutes, until the cauliflower is tender but not mushy.

7. Remove from heat and garnish with chopped fresh cilantro, if desired, before serving.

Tips/Notes:

Ensure the cauliflower rice is not overcrowded in the skillet to allow even cooking and prevent mushiness.

Customize your stir-fry by adding protein sources like diced chicken, shrimp, or tofu, if desired.

For additional flavor, sprinkle with sesame seeds or a squeeze of lime juice before serving.

Leftover cauliflower rice stir-fry can be stored in an airtight container in the refrigerator for up to 3 days.

Nutritional Information (per serving, based on 4 servings):

Calories: 120 kcal

Protein: 4g

Carbohydrates: 16g

Fiber: 6g

Fat: 6g

Saturated Fat: 3g

Cholesterol: 0mg

Sodium: 350mg

Potassium: 680mg

This Cauliflower "Rice" Stir Fry is a flavorful and nutrient-dense dish that adheres to the Anti-inflammatory Autoimmune Protocol (AIP) guidelines. It replaces traditional rice with cauliflower, providing a low-carb, gluten-free alternative packed with vitamins, minerals, and fiber from a variety of colorful vegetables. Enjoy this satisfying stir-fry as a main course or side dish, perfect for those seeking a delicious and inflammation-friendly meal option.

Stuffed Acorn Squash

Ingredients:
2 acorn squash, halved and seeds removed
1 tablespoon olive oil or avocado oil
1 onion, finely chopped
2 cloves garlic, minced
1 cup mushrooms, chopped
1 cup spinach, chopped
1/2 cup cooked quinoa (omit for strict AIP)
1/4 cup chopped walnuts or pecans (omit for strict AIP)
1 teaspoon dried thyme
Sea salt and freshly ground black pepper, to taste
Fresh parsley, chopped (optional, for garnish)

Instructions:
1. Preheat the oven to 400°F (200°C).
2. Cut the acorn squash in half and scoop out the seeds. Place the squash halves cut-side down on a baking sheet lined with parchment paper.
3. Bake the squash in the preheated oven for 30-35 minutes, or until tender when pierced with a fork.

4. While the squash is baking, heat olive oil or avocado oil in a large skillet over medium heat.

5. Add chopped onion and minced garlic to the skillet, sautéing until softened and fragrant.

6. Stir in chopped mushrooms and cook until mushrooms are tender and slightly browned.

7. Add chopped spinach, cooked quinoa (if using), chopped nuts (if using), dried thyme, sea salt, and freshly ground black pepper to the skillet. Cook until spinach is wilted and ingredients are well combined.

8. Remove the squash halves from the oven and carefully flip them over.

9. Spoon the quinoa and vegetable mixture evenly into each squash half.

10. Garnish with chopped fresh parsley, if desired, before serving.

Tips/Notes:
Customize the stuffing with other vegetables like bell peppers or zucchini.
For added protein, include cooked ground turkey or chicken (if tolerated).
Substitute nuts with toasted pumpkin seeds for an AIP-compliant alternative.
Leftover stuffed acorn squash can be stored in an airtight container in the refrigerator for up to 3 days.

Nutritional Information (per serving, based on 4 servings):
Calories: 250 kcal
Protein: 6g
Carbohydrates: 40g
Fiber: 6g
Fat: 10g
Saturated Fat: 1g

Cholesterol: 0mg
Sodium: 20mg
Potassium: 1000mg

This Stuffed Acorn Squash recipe offers a hearty and nutritious meal option that adheres to the Anti-inflammatory Autoimmune Protocol (AIP) guidelines. It combines the natural sweetness of acorn squash with a savory and flavorful stuffing of vegetables, nuts (optional), and herbs, providing a satisfying dish rich in vitamins, minerals, and dietary fiber. Enjoy this dish as a comforting main course or impressive side dish, perfect for sharing with family and friends.

Zucchini Noodles with Pesto

Ingredients:
4 medium zucchini, spiralized into noodles
1 cup fresh basil leaves
1/4 cup pine nuts
1/4 cup extra virgin olive oil
2 cloves garlic, minced
Juice of 1/2 lemon
Sea salt and freshly ground black pepper, to taste
Nutritional yeast (optional, for a cheesy flavor)

Instructions:
1. Spiralize the zucchini into noodles using a spiralizer. Set aside in a large mixing bowl.

2. In a food processor or blender, combine fresh basil leaves, pine nuts, extra virgin olive oil, minced garlic, lemon juice, sea salt, and freshly ground black pepper.

3. Blend until smooth and creamy, scraping down the sides as needed to ensure all ingredients are well combined.

4. Pour the pesto sauce over the zucchini noodles and toss gently to coat evenly.

5. Serve immediately, garnished with nutritional yeast (if using) for added flavor.

Tips/Notes:

Adjust the consistency of the pesto by adding more olive oil or a splash of water if needed.

For a nut-free version, substitute pine nuts with sunflower seeds or omit altogether.

Customize your zucchini noodles with additional toppings such as cherry tomatoes, sliced olives, or grilled chicken (if tolerated).

Leftover zucchini noodles with pesto can be stored in an airtight container in the refrigerator for up to 2 days.

Nutritional Information (per serving, based on 4 servings):

Calories: 200 kcal

Protein: 4g

Carbohydrates: 10g

Fiber: 3g

Fat: 17g

Saturated Fat: 2g

Cholesterol: 0mg

Sodium: 150mg

Potassium: 650mg

This Zucchini Noodles with Pesto recipe offers a fresh and vibrant dish that aligns with the Anti-inflammatory Autoimmune Protocol

(AIP) guidelines. It replaces traditional pasta with spiralized zucchini noodles and features a dairy-free pesto sauce made from fresh basil, pine nuts, and extra virgin olive oil. Enjoy this light and flavorful meal as a nutritious alternative to pasta, packed with vitamins, minerals, and healthy fats to support your health and well-being.

Sweet Potato and Avocado Salad

Ingredients:
2 medium sweet potatoes, peeled and diced
1 avocado, diced
1/4 cup red onion, finely chopped
1/4 cup fresh cilantro, chopped
Juice of 1 lime
2 tablespoons olive oil or avocado oil
Sea salt and freshly ground black pepper, to taste
Optional: chopped jalapeño for a spicy kick

Instructions:
1. Steam or boil diced sweet potatoes until tender but still firm. Drain and let cool.
2. In a large mixing bowl, combine diced avocado, finely chopped red onion, and fresh cilantro.
3. Add the cooled sweet potatoes to the bowl.
4. Drizzle lime juice and olive oil (or avocado oil) over the salad ingredients.
5. Gently toss to combine, ensuring the avocado coats the sweet potatoes evenly.
6. Season with sea salt and freshly ground black pepper to taste.

7. If desired, add chopped jalapeño for a spicy kick and additional flavor.

8. Serve immediately or refrigerate for 30 minutes to allow flavors to meld before serving.

Tips/Notes:

To save time, roast sweet potatoes instead of steaming or boiling for added depth of flavor.

Adjust the amount of lime juice and olive oil based on personal preference.

For added protein, include diced grilled chicken or tofu (if tolerated).

This salad is best enjoyed fresh but can be stored in an airtight container in the refrigerator for up to 2 days.

Nutritional Information (per serving, based on 4 servings):

Calories: 180 kcal

Protein: 3g

Carbohydrates: 20g

Fiber: 5g

Fat: 11g

Saturated Fat: 1.5g

Cholesterol: 0mg

Sodium: 80mg

Potassium: 580mg

This Sweet Potato and Avocado Salad is a refreshing and nutrient-dense dish that aligns with the Anti-inflammatory Autoimmune Protocol (AIP) guidelines. It combines the creamy texture of avocado with the sweetness of sweet potatoes, enhanced with fresh cilantro and lime juice for a vibrant flavor profile. Enjoy this salad as a satisfying side dish or light meal, perfect for those seeking a flavorful and health-conscious option that supports overall well-being.

Balsamic Glazed Brussels Sprouts

Ingredients:
1 lb Brussels sprouts, trimmed and halved
2 tablespoons balsamic vinegar
1 tablespoon olive oil or avocado oil
1 tablespoon honey (omit for strict AIP)
Sea salt and freshly ground black pepper, to taste
Optional: crushed red pepper flakes for a hint of spice

Instructions:
1. Preheat the oven to 400°F (200°C) and line a baking sheet with parchment paper.
2. In a large mixing bowl, combine Brussels sprouts, balsamic vinegar, olive oil or avocado oil, and honey (if using).
3. Toss Brussels sprouts until evenly coated with the mixture.
4. Arrange Brussels sprouts in a single layer on the prepared baking sheet, cut-side down.
5. Season with sea salt and freshly ground black pepper to taste. Add crushed red pepper flakes for a spicy kick, if desired.
6. Roast in the preheated oven for 20-25 minutes, stirring halfway through, until Brussels sprouts are tender and caramelized.
7. Remove from the oven and drizzle with additional balsamic vinegar before serving.

Tips/Notes:

For a vegan option, substitute honey with maple syrup or omit altogether.
Ensure Brussels sprouts are evenly coated with the balsamic mixture to enhance flavor.
Adjust roasting time based on desired level of caramelization.
Serve as a delicious side dish or appetizer, garnished with fresh herbs like parsley or thyme.

Nutritional Information (per serving, based on 4 servings):
Calories: 80 kcal
Protein: 3g
Carbohydrates: 12g
Fiber: 4g
Fat: 3g
Saturated Fat: 0g
Cholesterol: 0mg
Sodium: 20mg
Potassium: 480mg

These Balsamic Glazed Brussels Sprouts offer a flavorful and nutritious side dish that aligns with the Anti-inflammatory Autoimmune Protocol (AIP) guidelines. The natural sweetness of balsamic vinegar complements the roasted Brussels sprouts, creating a caramelized exterior while maintaining a tender texture. Enjoy this dish as a savory addition to any meal, providing essential vitamins, minerals, and dietary fiber to support overall health and well being.

Coconut Curry Butternut Squash Soup

Ingredients:

1 medium butternut squash, peeled, seeded, and diced

1 tablespoon coconut oil

1 onion, chopped

2 cloves garlic, minced

1 tablespoon grated ginger

1 tablespoon curry powder

1 can (14 oz) full-fat coconut milk

4 cups vegetable broth

Sea salt and freshly ground black pepper, to taste

Fresh cilantro, chopped (optional, for garnish)

Toasted coconut flakes (optional, for garnish)

Instructions:

1. In a large pot or Dutch oven, heat coconut oil over medium heat.

2. Add chopped onion and sauté until translucent, about 5 minutes.

3. Stir in minced garlic, grated ginger, and curry powder. Cook for another 1-2 minutes until fragrant.

4. Add diced butternut squash to the pot, stirring to coat with the spices and onion mixture.

5. Pour in coconut milk and vegetable broth, stirring well to combine.

6. Bring the soup to a boil, then reduce heat and simmer uncovered for 20-25 minutes, or until butternut squash is tender.

7. Remove from heat and let the soup cool slightly.

8. Using an immersion blender or regular blender, puree the soup until smooth and creamy.

9. Season with sea salt and freshly ground black pepper to taste.

10. Serve hot, garnished with chopped fresh cilantro and toasted coconut flakes, if desired.

Tips/Notes:

To save time, use pre-cut butternut squash cubes or puree.

Adjust the consistency of the soup by adding more vegetable broth or coconut milk as needed.

For added protein, stir in cooked shredded chicken or chickpeas (if tolerated).

Store leftover soup in an airtight container in the refrigerator for up to 4 days or freeze for longer storage.

Nutritional Information (per serving, based on 6 servings):

Calories: 220 kcal

Protein: 3g

Carbohydrates: 20g

Fiber: 4g

Fat: 15g

Saturated Fat: 13g

Cholesterol: 0mg

Sodium: 600mg

Potassium: 600mg

This Coconut Curry Butternut Squash Soup is a comforting and nourishing dish that adheres to the Anti-inflammatory Autoimmune Protocol (AIP) guidelines. It combines the creamy texture of coconut milk with the warmth of curry spices, complemented by the sweetness of butternut squash. Enjoy this flavorful soup as a wholesome meal option, providing essential nutrients and anti-inflammatory benefits to support overall health and well-being.

Garlic and Herb Roasted Mushrooms

Ingredients:
1 lb mushrooms (such as cremini or button), cleaned and halved
3 tablespoons olive oil
4 cloves garlic, minced
1 tablespoon fresh thyme leaves
1 tablespoon fresh rosemary, chopped
Sea salt and freshly ground black pepper, to taste
Fresh parsley, chopped (optional, for garnish)

Instructions:
1. Preheat the oven to 400°F (200°C) and line a baking sheet with parchment paper.
2. In a large mixing bowl, combine halved mushrooms, olive oil, minced garlic, fresh thyme leaves, and chopped rosemary.
3. Toss the mushrooms until evenly coated with the olive oil and herbs.
4. Season with sea salt and freshly ground black pepper to taste.
5. Spread the mushrooms in a single layer on the prepared baking sheet.
6. Roast in the preheated oven for 20-25 minutes, stirring halfway through, until mushrooms are tender and golden brown.
7. Remove from the oven and garnish with chopped fresh parsley, if desired, before serving.

Tips/Notes:

Choose mushrooms that are firm and evenly sized for even roasting.

For a richer flavor, add a drizzle of balsamic vinegar or sprinkle with nutritional yeast before roasting.

Serve as a side dish, over pasta, or as a topping for grilled meats or salads.

Leftover roasted mushrooms can be stored in an airtight container in the refrigerator for up to 3 days.

Nutritional Information (per serving, based on 4 servings):
Calories: 120 kcal
Protein: 3g
Carbohydrates: 6g
Fiber: 2g
Fat: 10g
Saturated Fat: 1.5g
Cholesterol: 0mg
Sodium: 10mg
Potassium: 420mg

These Garlic and Herb Roasted Mushrooms are a savory and aromatic dish that fits well with the Anti-inflammatory Autoimmune Protocol (AIP) guidelines. They're simple to prepare yet packed with flavor from fresh herbs and garlic, making them a versatile addition to any meal. Enjoy these roasted mushrooms as a delicious side dish or incorporate them into various recipes for added depth and earthy richness.

Carrot Ginger Soup

Ingredients:
1 lb carrots, peeled and chopped
1 onion, chopped
2 cloves garlic, minced
1 tablespoon fresh ginger, grated
4 cups vegetable broth
1 cup full-fat coconut milk
2 tablespoons olive oil or avocado oil
Sea salt and freshly ground black pepper, to taste
Fresh cilantro, chopped (optional, for garnish)

Instructions:
1. In a large pot or Dutch oven, heat olive oil or avocado oil over medium heat.
2. Add chopped onion and sauté until translucent, about 5 minutes.
3. Stir in minced garlic and grated ginger, cooking for another 1-2 minutes until fragrant.
4. Add chopped carrots to the pot, stirring to coat with the onion mixture.
5. Pour in vegetable broth, bring to a boil, then reduce heat and simmer uncovered for 20-25 minutes, or until carrots are tender.
6. Remove from heat and let the soup cool slightly.
7. Using an immersion blender or regular blender, puree the soup until smooth and creamy.
8. Stir in coconut milk, and season with sea salt and freshly ground black pepper to taste.

9. Return the soup to low heat, simmer for an additional 5 minutes to heat through.
10. Serve hot, garnished with chopped fresh cilantro, if desired.

Tips/Notes:
For added flavor, roast carrots before adding them to the soup.
Adjust the consistency of the soup by adding more vegetable broth or coconut milk as needed.
Garnish with a drizzle of coconut milk or a sprinkle of ground cinnamon for an extra touch of flavor.
Store leftover soup in an airtight container in the refrigerator for up to 4 days or freeze for longer storage.

Nutritional Information (per serving, based on 6 servings):
Calories: 180 kcal
Protein: 3g
Carbohydrates: 16g
Fiber: 4g
Fat: 12g
Saturated Fat: 7g
Cholesterol: 0mg
Sodium: 600mg
Potassium: 600mg

This Carrot Ginger Soup is a comforting and nourishing dish that aligns with the Anti-inflammatory Autoimmune Protocol (AIP) guidelines. It combines the natural sweetness of carrots with the warmth of fresh ginger and the creaminess of coconut milk, creating a flavorful and satisfying soup. Enjoy this nutrient-dense soup as a light meal or appetizer, providing essential vitamins, minerals, and antioxidants to support overall health and well-being.

Spaghetti Squash Primavera

Ingredients:
1 medium spaghetti squash
2 tablespoons olive oil or avocado oil
1 onion, thinly sliced
2 cloves garlic, minced
1 red bell pepper, thinly sliced
1 yellow bell pepper, thinly sliced
1 zucchini, thinly sliced
1 cup cherry tomatoes, halved
1/2 cup vegetable broth
1 tablespoon fresh basil, chopped
Sea salt and freshly ground black pepper, to taste
Optional: grated dairy-free cheese (omit for strict AIP)

Instructions:
1. Preheat the oven to 400°F (200°C).
2. Cut the spaghetti squash in half lengthwise and scoop out the seeds.
3. Brush the cut sides with olive oil or avocado oil and place them cut-side down on a baking sheet lined with parchment paper.
4. Roast the spaghetti squash in the preheated oven for 40-50 minutes, or until tender and easily pierced with a fork.
5. While the squash is roasting, heat 1 tablespoon of olive oil or avocado oil in a large skillet over medium heat.
6. Add thinly sliced onion and minced garlic to the skillet, sautéing until softened and fragrant.

7. Stir in thinly sliced red and yellow bell peppers, zucchini, and cherry tomatoes. Cook for 5-7 minutes, until vegetables are tender-crisp.

8. Add vegetable broth to the skillet and simmer for another 2-3 minutes.

9. Once the spaghetti squash is cooked, use a fork to scrape the flesh into strands.

10. Add the spaghetti squash strands to the skillet with the cooked vegetables.

11. Drizzle with the remaining tablespoon of olive oil or avocado oil, and sprinkle with chopped fresh basil.

12. Season with sea salt and freshly ground black pepper to taste, tossing gently to combine.

13. Serve hot, optionally garnished with grated dairy-free cheese if desired.

Tips/Notes:

Customize the primavera with your favorite seasonal vegetables. For added protein, toss in cooked chicken, shrimp, or tofu (if tolerated).

Store leftover spaghetti squash primavera in an airtight container in the refrigerator for up to 3 days.

Nutritional Information (per serving, based on 4 servings):
Calories: 180 kcal
Protein: 3g
Carbohydrates: 24g
Fiber: 5g
Fat: 9g
Saturated Fat: 1g
Cholesterol: 0mg
Sodium: 240mg
Potassium: 700mg

This Spaghetti Squash Primavera is a delicious and vibrant dish that aligns with the Anti-inflammatory Autoimmune Protocol (AIP) guidelines. It replaces traditional pasta with spaghetti squash, offering a gluten-free and nutrient-dense alternative. Enjoy this colorful and flavorful meal as a wholesome option packed with vitamins, minerals, and antioxidants to support your health and well-being.

Beet and Carrot Slaw

Ingredients:
2 medium beets, peeled and grated
2 large carrots, peeled and grated
1/4 cup fresh parsley, chopped
1/4 cup fresh cilantro, chopped
2 tablespoons apple cider vinegar
1 tablespoon olive oil
1 tablespoon honey (omit for strict AIP)
Sea salt and freshly ground black pepper, to taste
Optional: toasted sesame seeds for garnish

Instructions:
1. In a large mixing bowl, combine grated beets and carrots.
2. Add chopped fresh parsley and cilantro to the bowl.
3. In a small bowl, whisk together apple cider vinegar, olive oil, and honey (if using).
4. Pour the dressing over the vegetables and herbs, tossing gently to coat evenly.
5. Season with sea salt and freshly ground black pepper to taste.

6. Cover and refrigerate the slaw for at least 30 minutes to allow flavors to meld.

7. Before serving, toss the slaw again and adjust seasoning if necessary.

8. Garnish with toasted sesame seeds, if desired.

Tips/Notes:

Use a box grater or food processor with a grating attachment to grate the beets and carrots quickly.

For a tangier slaw, increase the amount of apple cider vinegar or add a splash of lemon juice.

Replace honey with maple syrup or omit altogether for a stricter AIP version.

Serve as a refreshing side dish or topping for burgers, tacos, or wraps.

Nutritional Information (per serving, based on 4 servings):

Calories: 90 kcal

Protein: 2g

Carbohydrates: 14g

Fiber: 4g

Fat: 4g

Saturated Fat: 0.5g

Cholesterol: 0mg

Sodium: 90mg

Potassium: 450mg

This Beet and Carrot Slaw is a vibrant and nutrient-packed dish that aligns with the Anti-inflammatory Autoimmune Protocol (AIP) guidelines. It combines the earthy sweetness of beets and carrots with fresh herbs and a tangy dressing, creating a flavorful and refreshing slaw. Enjoy this colorful salad as a nutritious addition to your meals, providing essential vitamins, minerals, and antioxidants to support overall health and well-being.

Avocado Cucumber Gazpacho

Ingredients:
2 ripe avocados, peeled and pitted
2 cucumbers, peeled and chopped
1 green bell pepper, chopped
1/2 red onion, chopped
2 cloves garlic, minced
2 cups vegetable broth
1/4 cup fresh cilantro, chopped
Juice of 1 lime
2 tablespoons olive oil
Sea salt and freshly ground black pepper, to taste
Optional: diced tomatoes and additional cilantro for garnish

Instructions:
1. In a blender or food processor, combine ripe avocados, chopped cucumbers, chopped green bell pepper, chopped red onion, minced garlic, vegetable broth, fresh cilantro, lime juice, and olive oil.
2. Blend until smooth and creamy, adjusting the consistency with additional vegetable broth if needed.
3. Season with sea salt and freshly ground black pepper to taste.
4. Transfer the gazpacho to a large mixing bowl and refrigerate for at least 1 hour to chill.
5. Before serving, stir the gazpacho well and adjust seasoning if necessary.

6. Serve chilled, garnished with diced tomatoes and additional chopped cilantro if desired.

Tips/Notes:
For a smoother texture, strain the gazpacho through a fine mesh sieve before chilling.
Customize with your favorite herbs such as parsley or basil for added flavor.
Adjust the lime juice and sea salt to balance the flavors according to your preference.
Store leftover gazpacho in an airtight container in the refrigerator for up to 3 days.

Nutritional Information (per serving, based on 4 servings):
Calories: 220 kcal
Protein: 4g
Carbohydrates: 16g
Fiber: 8g
Fat: 18g
Saturated Fat: 3g
Cholesterol: 0mg
Sodium: 480mg
Potassium: 900mg

This Avocado Cucumber Gazpacho is a refreshing and nutritious soup that aligns with the Anti-inflammatory Autoimmune Protocol (AIP) guidelines. It combines creamy avocado with crisp cucumber and a blend of fresh vegetables, creating a cooling and satisfying dish perfect for warm weather. Enjoy this gazpacho as a light appetizer or meal, providing essential vitamins, minerals, and healthy fats to support your health and well-being.

V

Poultry, Meat and Protein

Introducing poultry into an Anti-inflammatory Autoimmune Protocol (AIP) diet can provide a versatile source of lean protein that aligns with the protocol's guidelines. Poultry, such as chicken and turkey, is often well-tolerated and can be prepared in various ways to suit different tastes and dietary needs.

Chicken and turkey are rich in essential nutrients like protein, B vitamins, and minerals such as zinc and selenium, which are crucial for immune function and overall health. When preparing poultry on the AIP diet, it's important to avoid inflammatory ingredients like processed sauces, refined oils, and excessive amounts of spices or seasonings that may trigger autoimmune responses in some individuals.

Opting for organic, pasture-raised poultry ensures higher quality meat with fewer contaminants and a better nutrient profile. Simple cooking methods like baking, grilling, or simmering with AIP-approved herbs and seasonings can enhance flavor without compromising dietary restrictions. Incorporating poultry into soups, salads, stir-fries, and roasted dishes allows for a diverse range of meal options that support healing and inflammation reduction.

Overall, poultry serves as a valuable component of the AIP diet, offering nourishing protein and essential nutrients while adhering to the protocol's principles of promoting gut health, reducing inflammation, and supporting immune function.

Lemon Herb Roasted Chicken

Ingredients:
1 whole chicken (about 3-4 lbs), giblets removed
2 lemons, divided
4 cloves garlic, minced
2 tablespoons fresh rosemary, chopped
2 tablespoons fresh thyme leaves
1/4 cup olive oil or avocado oil
Sea salt and freshly ground black pepper, to taste
Fresh parsley, chopped (optional, for garnish)

Instructions:
1. Preheat the oven to 425°F (220°C).
2. Rinse the chicken under cold water and pat dry with paper towels.
3. Zest and juice one lemon. Cut the other lemon into wedges.
4. In a small bowl, combine minced garlic, chopped rosemary, chopped thyme, lemon zest, lemon juice, and olive oil.
5. Season the chicken cavity with sea salt and freshly ground black pepper.

6. Place the lemon wedges inside the cavity of the chicken.

7. Rub the herb mixture all over the chicken, ensuring it's evenly coated.

8. Tie the legs together with kitchen twine and tuck the wing tips under the body of the chicken.

9. Place the chicken breast-side up on a rack in a roasting pan.

10. Roast the chicken in the preheated oven for 1 hour to 1 hour 15 minutes, or until the internal temperature reaches 165°F (75°C) and the juices run clear.

11. Remove from the oven and let the chicken rest for 10 minutes before carving.

12. Garnish with chopped fresh parsley before serving.

Tips/Notes:

For a crispier skin, pat the chicken dry and let it air dry in the refrigerator uncovered for a few hours or overnight before roasting.

Ensure the chicken is fully cooked by checking the internal temperature with a meat thermometer.

Serve with roasted vegetables or a fresh salad for a complete meal.

Leftover chicken can be used in soups, salads, or sandwiches.

Nutritional Information (per serving, based on 4 servings):

Calories: 400 kcal

Protein: 32g

Carbohydrates: 4g

Fiber: 1g

Fat: 29g

Saturated Fat: 6g

Cholesterol: 120mg

Sodium: 110mg

Potassium: 380mg

This Lemon Herb Roasted Chicken is a classic dish that fits well within the Anti-inflammatory Autoimmune Protocol (AIP) guidelines. It's seasoned with fresh herbs and lemon, providing a burst of flavor without compromising dietary restrictions. Enjoy this tender and juicy roasted chicken as a comforting and nourishing meal, perfect for family dinners or special occasions.

AIP Chicken Tenders

Ingredients:

1 lb chicken breast tenders, cut into strips

1/2 cup coconut flour

1 teaspoon garlic powder

1 teaspoon onion powder

1 teaspoon dried thyme

1/2 teaspoon sea salt

1/4 teaspoon freshly ground black pepper (omit for strict AIP)

2 tablespoons coconut oil or avocado oil, for frying

Instructions:

1. In a shallow bowl or plate, combine coconut flour, garlic powder, onion powder, dried thyme, sea salt, and black pepper (if using).

2. Heat coconut oil or avocado oil in a large skillet over medium heat.

3. Dredge each chicken tender in the coconut flour mixture, shaking off any excess.

4. Place the coated chicken tenders in the heated skillet, ensuring they are not overcrowded.

5. Cook for 4-5 minutes per side, or until golden brown and cooked through.

6. Remove chicken tenders from the skillet and place on a plate lined with paper towels to absorb excess oil.

7. Serve hot with your favorite AIP-friendly dipping sauce or alongside roasted vegetables.

Tips/Notes:

Ensure the skillet is adequately heated before adding the chicken tenders to achieve a crispy exterior.

For additional flavor, add AIP-approved herbs or spices to the coconut flour mixture.

Use tongs to carefully flip the chicken tenders to prevent them from breaking apart.

Leftover chicken tenders can be stored in an airtight container in the refrigerator for up to 3 days.

Nutritional Information (per serving, based on 4 servings):

Calories: 250 kcal

Protein: 28g

Carbohydrates: 8g

Fiber: 4g

Fat: 12g

Saturated Fat: 7g

Cholesterol: 75mg

Sodium: 350mg

Potassium: 420mg

These AIP Chicken Tenders are a delicious and satisfying option that adheres to the Anti-inflammatory Autoimmune Protocol (AIP) guidelines. They are coated in coconut flour and seasoned with AIP-friendly herbs and spices, providing a crunchy exterior and tender interior without grains or dairy. Enjoy these chicken tenders as a flavorful main dish or appetizer, perfect for those following a restricted diet due to autoimmune conditions or seeking a healthier alternative to traditional fried foods.

Turmeric Chicken Skewers

Ingredients:
1 lb chicken breast, cut into cubes
1 tablespoon olive oil or avocado oil
2 teaspoons ground turmeric
1 teaspoon ground cumin
1/2 teaspoon ground ginger
1/2 teaspoon sea salt
1/4 teaspoon freshly ground black pepper (omit for strict AIP)
Wooden skewers, soaked in water for 30 minutes

Instructions:
1. In a bowl, combine olive oil or avocado oil, ground turmeric, ground cumin, ground ginger, sea salt, and black pepper (if using).
2. Add the cubed chicken breast to the bowl, tossing to coat evenly with the spice mixture. Marinate for at least 30 minutes in the refrigerator.
3. Preheat the grill or grill pan over medium-high heat.
4. Thread the marinated chicken cubes onto the soaked wooden skewers, leaving a little space between each piece.
5. Grill the chicken skewers for 4-5 minutes on each side, or until fully cooked through and grill marks appear.
6. Remove from the grill and let the skewers rest for a few minutes before serving.

Tips/Notes:

Adjust the amount of spices according to your taste preferences.

If using wooden skewers, remember to soak them in water for at least 30 minutes to prevent burning on the grill.

Serve with a side of AIP-approved vegetables or a fresh salad for a complete meal.

Leftover skewers can be refrigerated and enjoyed cold or reheated briefly in the oven.

Nutritional Information (per serving, based on 4 servings):

Calories: 180 kcal

Protein: 25g

Carbohydrates: 1g

Fiber: 0g

Fat: 8g

Saturated Fat: 1g

Cholesterol: 75mg

Sodium: 300mg

Potassium: 350mg

These Turmeric Chicken Skewers are a flavorful and nutritious dish that fits within the Anti-inflammatory Autoimmune Protocol (AIP) guidelines. Turmeric, cumin, and ginger provide anti-inflammatory properties while enhancing the taste of the grilled chicken. Enjoy these skewers as a protein-rich main dish, perfect for summer barbecues or any time you crave a delicious and health-conscious meal.

Herbed Chicken Salad

Ingredients:
1 lb chicken breast, cooked and shredded
1/2 cup celery, finely chopped
1/4 cup red onion, finely chopped
1/4 cup fresh parsley, chopped
2 tablespoons fresh dill, chopped
1/2 cup AIP-friendly mayonnaise (homemade or store-bought)
1 tablespoon apple cider vinegar
Sea salt and freshly ground black pepper, to taste (omit black pepper for strict AIP)

Instructions:
1. In a large mixing bowl, combine shredded chicken breast, chopped celery, chopped red onion, chopped parsley, and chopped dill.
2. In a small bowl, whisk together AIP-friendly mayonnaise and apple cider vinegar until well combined.
3. Pour the dressing over the chicken mixture, tossing gently to coat evenly.
4. Season with sea salt and freshly ground black pepper to taste (omit black pepper for strict AIP).
5. Cover the bowl and refrigerate the chicken salad for at least 30 minutes to allow flavors to meld.
6. Before serving, toss the chicken salad again and adjust seasoning if necessary.
7. Serve chilled on a bed of lettuce, in lettuce wraps, or with gluten-free crackers.

Tips/Notes:

Use cooked and cooled chicken for best results in this salad.

Customize with additional herbs like basil or chives for added flavor.

Serve as a light meal, sandwich filling, or appetizer.

Store leftover chicken salad in an airtight container in the refrigerator for up to 3 days.

Nutritional Information (per serving, based on 4 servings):

Calories: 250 kcal

Protein: 25g

Carbohydrates: 3g

Fiber: 1g

Fat: 15g

Saturated Fat: 2g

Cholesterol: 75mg

Sodium: 250mg

Potassium: 300mg

This Herbed Chicken Salad is a refreshing and satisfying dish that aligns with the Anti-inflammatory Autoimmune Protocol (AIP) guidelines. It combines tender shredded chicken with fresh herbs and a creamy, tangy dressing, providing a balanced and nutrient-dense meal option. Enjoy this versatile chicken salad as a healthy lunch or dinner choice, offering protein, healthy fats, and essential vitamins to support overall health and well-being.

Baked Chicken Thighs with Rosemary

Ingredients:

4 chicken thighs, bone-in and skin-on
2 tablespoons olive oil or avocado oil
2 cloves garlic, minced
1 tablespoon fresh rosemary, chopped
Sea salt and freshly ground black pepper, to taste (omit black pepper for strict AIP)

Instructions:
1. Preheat the oven to 400°F (200°C).
2. In a small bowl, combine olive oil or avocado oil, minced garlic, chopped fresh rosemary, sea salt, and freshly ground black pepper (if using).
3. Place the chicken thighs on a baking sheet lined with parchment paper or in a baking dish.
4. Rub the herb mixture evenly over the chicken thighs, ensuring they are well coated.
5. Arrange the chicken thighs skin-side up on the baking sheet or dish.
6. Bake in the preheated oven for 30-35 minutes, or until the chicken thighs are golden brown and cooked through, with an internal temperature of 165°F (75°C).
7. Remove from the oven and let the chicken thighs rest for a few minutes before serving.

Tips/Notes:
Adjust baking time depending on the size and thickness of the chicken thighs.
For crispier skin, broil the chicken thighs for an additional 2-3 minutes after baking.
Serve with roasted vegetables or a side salad for a complete meal.
Leftover chicken thighs can be stored in an airtight container in the refrigerator for up to 3 days.

Nutritional Information (per serving, based on 4 servings):
Calories: 300 kcal
Protein: 25g
Carbohydrates: 0g
Fiber: 0g
Fat: 22g
Saturated Fat: 5g
Cholesterol: 140mg
Sodium: 350mg
Potassium: 280mg

These Baked Chicken Thighs with Rosemary are a simple yet flavorful dish that adheres to the Anti-inflammatory Autoimmune Protocol (AIP) guidelines. The combination of fresh rosemary and garlic enhances the natural flavors of the chicken thighs, creating a delicious and comforting meal option. Enjoy these tender and juicy chicken thighs as a versatile main dish, perfect for weeknight dinners or special occasions.

AIP Chicken and Vegetable Soup

Ingredients:
1 lb chicken breast or thighs, boneless and skinless, cut into bite-sized pieces
4 cups chicken broth, homemade or low-sodium store-bought
2 carrots, peeled and diced
2 celery stalks, diced
1 medium sweet potato, peeled and diced
1/2 onion, diced
2 cloves garlic, minced

1 teaspoon fresh ginger, grated
1 teaspoon dried thyme
1/2 teaspoon dried oregano
Sea salt and freshly ground black pepper, to taste (omit black pepper for strict AIP)
2 tablespoons fresh parsley, chopped (for garnish)
Optional: additional vegetables such as spinach or kale

Instructions:
1. In a large pot or Dutch oven, heat olive oil or avocado oil over medium heat.
2. Add diced onion and minced garlic, sautéing until fragrant and translucent, about 3-4 minutes.
3. Add diced carrots, celery, and sweet potato to the pot, stirring to combine with the onions and garlic.
4. Pour in chicken broth and bring to a boil. Reduce heat to low and let simmer for 10-15 minutes, or until vegetables are tender.
5. Add diced chicken pieces, grated ginger, dried thyme, and dried oregano to the pot. Simmer for an additional 10-15 minutes, or until chicken is cooked through.
6. Season with sea salt and freshly ground black pepper to taste (omit black pepper for strict AIP).
7. Remove from heat and garnish with chopped fresh parsley before serving.
8. Serve hot as a comforting and nourishing meal.

Tips/Notes:
Customize the soup with additional AIP-approved vegetables such as spinach or kale.
Make a larger batch and freeze individual portions for quick and convenient meals.
Substitute chicken breast with chicken thighs or shredded leftover chicken for variation.

Adjust cooking time depending on the size and thickness of chicken pieces.

Nutritional Information (per serving, based on 4 servings):
Calories: 250 kcal
Protein: 25g
Carbohydrates: 20g
Fiber: 4g
Fat: 8g
Saturated Fat: 2g
Cholesterol: 60mg
Sodium: 600mg
Potassium: 800mg

This AIP Chicken and Vegetable Soup is a hearty and nutritious dish that aligns with the Anti-inflammatory Autoimmune Protocol (AIP) guidelines. It combines tender chicken with a variety of vegetables and aromatic herbs, providing a comforting and satisfying meal option. Enjoy this flavorful soup as a nourishing lunch or dinner, packed with essential vitamins, minerals, and protein to support overall health and well-being.

Ginger-Lime Chicken Wings

Ingredients:
2 lbs chicken wings, tips removed and wings separated into drumettes and flats
2 tablespoons olive oil or avocado oil
Zest and juice of 1 lime
2 tablespoons coconut aminos

1 tablespoon fresh ginger, grated
2 cloves garlic, minced
1 tablespoon honey (optional, omit for strict AIP)
Sea salt and freshly ground black pepper, to taste (omit black pepper for strict AIP)
Fresh cilantro, chopped (for garnish)

Instructions:
1. Preheat the oven to 400°F (200°C).
2. In a bowl, whisk together olive oil or avocado oil, lime zest, lime juice, coconut aminos, grated ginger, minced garlic, honey (if using), sea salt, and freshly ground black pepper (if using).
3. Place the chicken wings in a large resealable plastic bag or a shallow dish.
4. Pour the marinade over the chicken wings, ensuring they are evenly coated. Marinate in the refrigerator for at least 30 minutes, or up to 2 hours for best flavor.
5. Line a baking sheet with parchment paper and arrange the chicken wings in a single layer.
6. Bake in the preheated oven for 40-45 minutes, turning halfway through, or until the wings are golden brown and crispy.
7. Remove from the oven and let the wings rest for a few minutes before serving.
8. Garnish with chopped fresh cilantro before serving.

Tips/Notes:
For extra crispy wings, broil for an additional 2-3 minutes after baking.
Adjust the amount of honey or omit entirely based on your sweetness preference.
Serve with a side of AIP-friendly vegetables or a fresh salad.
Leftover wings can be stored in an airtight container in the refrigerator for up to 3 days.

Nutritional Information (per serving, based on 4 servings):
Calories: 300 kcal
Protein: 20g
Carbohydrates: 5g
Fiber: 0g
Fat: 22g
Saturated Fat: 5g
Cholesterol: 80mg
Sodium: 350mg
Potassium: 250mg

These Ginger-Lime Chicken Wings are a flavorful and satisfying dish that adheres to the Anti-inflammatory Autoimmune Protocol (AIP) guidelines. The combination of fresh lime, ginger, and coconut aminos adds zesty and aromatic flavors to the crispy chicken wings, making them perfect for gatherings or as a delicious appetizer. Enjoy these wings as a healthier alternative to traditional fried wings, providing protein and essential nutrients while supporting a balanced and nutritious diet.

Coconut Milk Chicken Curry

Ingredients:
1 lb chicken breast or thighs, boneless and skinless, cut into bite-sized pieces
1 tablespoon coconut oil or avocado oil
1 onion, finely chopped
3 cloves garlic, minced
1 tablespoon fresh ginger, grated
1 tablespoon curry powder

1 teaspoon ground turmeric
1 can (14 oz) coconut milk
1 cup chicken broth, homemade or low-sodium store-bought
2 carrots, peeled and sliced
1 bell pepper, diced
1 cup broccoli florets
Sea salt, to taste
Fresh cilantro, chopped (for garnish)

Instructions:
1. In a large skillet or Dutch oven, heat coconut oil or avocado oil over medium heat.
2. Add chopped onion and sauté until translucent, about 4-5 minutes.
3. Add minced garlic and grated ginger, stirring constantly for another minute until fragrant.
4. Stir in curry powder and ground turmeric, cooking for 1 minute to toast the spices.
5. Add chicken pieces to the skillet, stirring to coat with the spice mixture, and cook until chicken is browned on all sides, about 5-6 minutes.
6. Pour in coconut milk and chicken broth, stirring well to combine. Bring to a simmer.
7. Add sliced carrots, diced bell pepper, and broccoli florets to the skillet. Cover and simmer over medium-low heat for 15-20 minutes, or until chicken is cooked through and vegetables are tender.
8. Season with sea salt to taste.
9. Garnish with chopped fresh cilantro before serving.

Tips/Notes:
Adjust the amount of curry powder and turmeric to suit your taste preferences.

Add additional vegetables such as spinach or zucchini for extra nutrition.

Serve the coconut milk chicken curry over cauliflower rice or with gluten-free noodles for a complete meal.

Store leftovers in an airtight container in the refrigerator for up to 3 days.

Nutritional Information (per serving, based on 4 servings):
Calories: 350 kcal
Protein: 25g
Carbohydrates: 12g
Fiber: 3g
Fat: 24g
Saturated Fat: 18g
Cholesterol: 70mg
Sodium: 400mg
Potassium: 800mg

This Coconut Milk Chicken Curry is a flavorful and creamy dish that complies with the Anti-inflammatory Autoimmune Protocol (AIP) guidelines. It combines tender chicken with aromatic spices and nutritious vegetables in a rich coconut milk base, offering a satisfying and nourishing meal option. Enjoy this comforting curry as a wholesome dinner choice, providing essential nutrients and vibrant flavors to support overall well-being.

Chicken and Broccoli Stir Fry

Ingredients:
1 lb chicken breast or thighs, boneless and skinless, thinly sliced
2 tablespoons coconut aminos

1 tablespoon arrowroot powder

2 tablespoons coconut oil or avocado oil

3 cloves garlic, minced

1 tablespoon fresh ginger, grated

1 head broccoli, cut into florets

1 bell pepper, sliced

1 carrot, thinly sliced

Sea salt and freshly ground black pepper, to taste (omit black pepper for strict AIP)

Fresh cilantro or green onions, chopped (for garnish)

Instructions:

1. In a bowl, combine sliced chicken breast or thighs with coconut aminos and arrowroot powder, tossing to coat evenly. Set aside to marinate for 10-15 minutes.

2. Heat coconut oil or avocado oil in a large skillet or wok over medium-high heat.

3. Add minced garlic and grated ginger to the skillet, stirring constantly for about 1 minute until fragrant.

4. Add marinated chicken to the skillet, spreading it into a single layer. Cook for 5-6 minutes, stirring occasionally, until chicken is browned and cooked through.

5. Add broccoli florets, sliced bell pepper, and carrot to the skillet, stirring to combine with the chicken. Cook for another 3-4 minutes, or until vegetables are tender-crisp.

6. Season with sea salt and freshly ground black pepper to taste (omit black pepper for strict AIP).

7. Remove from heat and garnish with chopped fresh cilantro or green onions before serving.

Tips/Notes:

Customize the stir fry with additional AIP-friendly vegetables such as mushrooms or snap peas.

Serve over cauliflower rice or with gluten-free noodles for a complete meal.
Substitute chicken with thinly sliced pork or beef for variation.
Store leftovers in an airtight container in the refrigerator for up to 3 days.

Nutritional Information (per serving, based on 4 servings):
Calories: 250 kcal
Protein: 25g
Carbohydrates: 12g
Fiber: 4g
Fat: 12g
Saturated Fat: 6g
Cholesterol: 70mg
Sodium: 300mg
Potassium: 800mg

This Chicken and Broccoli Stir Fry is a quick and nutritious dish that fits within the Anti-inflammatory Autoimmune Protocol (AIP) guidelines. It combines tender chicken with an array of colorful vegetables in a savory coconut aminos sauce, offering a balanced and flavorful meal option. Enjoy this stir fry as a satisfying lunch or dinner choice, providing protein, vitamins, and minerals to support a healthy lifestyle.

Stuffed Chicken Breasts with Spinach and Mushrooms

Ingredients:
4 chicken breasts, boneless and skinless
2 cups fresh spinach leaves
1 cup mushrooms, sliced
2 cloves garlic, minced
1 tablespoon olive oil or avocado oil
Sea salt and freshly ground black pepper, to taste (omit black pepper for strict AIP)
Toothpicks or kitchen twine

Instructions:
1. Preheat the oven to 375°F (190°C).
2. In a large skillet, heat olive oil or avocado oil over medium heat.
3. Add minced garlic and sauté for 1 minute until fragrant.
4. Add sliced mushrooms to the skillet and cook for 3-4 minutes until softened.
5. Add fresh spinach leaves to the skillet and cook until wilted, about 2-3 minutes. Season with sea salt and freshly ground black pepper to taste (omit black pepper for strict AIP).
6. Remove skillet from heat and let the spinach-mushroom mixture cool slightly.
7. Place each chicken breast between two sheets of plastic wrap or parchment paper. Use a meat mallet or rolling pin to pound the chicken breasts to an even thickness.

8. Spoon the spinach-mushroom mixture evenly onto each chicken breast.

9. Roll up each chicken breast tightly and secure with toothpicks or kitchen twine.

10. Place the stuffed chicken breasts in a baking dish lined with parchment paper.

11. Bake in the preheated oven for 25-30 minutes, or until chicken is cooked through and juices run clear.

12. Remove toothpicks or twine before serving.

Tips/Notes:

Feel free to add AIP-friendly herbs or spices to the spinach-mushroom mixture for added flavor.

Serve the stuffed chicken breasts with roasted vegetables or a side salad.

Ensure the chicken breasts are properly sealed to prevent filling from leaking during baking.

Store leftovers in an airtight container in the refrigerator for up to 3 days.

Nutritional Information (per serving, based on 4 servings):
Calories: 250 kcal
Protein: 35g
Carbohydrates: 4g
Fiber: 1g
Fat: 10g
Saturated Fat: 2g
Cholesterol: 100mg
Sodium: 300mg
Potassium: 600mg

These Stuffed Chicken Breasts with Spinach and Mushrooms are a delicious and nutritious option that aligns with the Anti-inflammatory Autoimmune Protocol (AIP) guidelines. The combination of tender chicken, flavorful spinach, and mushrooms creates a satisfying meal packed with protein and essential nutrients. Enjoy this dish as a wholesome dinner choice, offering a balance of flavors and textures to delight your taste buds.

Honey-Garlic Chicken Drumsticks

Ingredients:
8 chicken drumsticks
1/4 cup coconut aminos
2 tablespoons honey (optional, omit for strict AIP)
3 cloves garlic, minced
1 tablespoon apple cider vinegar
1 tablespoon olive oil or avocado oil
Sea salt and freshly ground black pepper, to taste (omit black pepper for strict AIP)
Fresh parsley or green onions, chopped (for garnish)

Instructions:
1. In a bowl, combine coconut aminos, honey (if using), minced garlic, apple cider vinegar, olive oil or avocado oil, sea salt, and freshly ground black pepper (if using).
2. Place chicken drumsticks in a large resealable plastic bag or shallow dish. Pour the marinade over the drumsticks, ensuring they are evenly coated. Marinate in the refrigerator for at least 30 minutes, or up to 2 hours for best flavor.
3. Preheat the oven to 400°F (200°C). Line a baking sheet with parchment paper.

4. Arrange marinated chicken drumsticks on the prepared baking sheet in a single layer.

5. Bake in the preheated oven for 35-40 minutes, turning halfway through, or until chicken is cooked through and juices run clear.

6. Remove from the oven and let the drumsticks rest for a few minutes before serving.

7. Garnish with chopped fresh parsley or green onions before serving.

Tips/Notes:

For a deeper flavor, you can marinate the drumsticks overnight in the refrigerator.

Adjust honey quantity based on your sweetness preference or omit entirely for strict AIP.

Serve with roasted vegetables or a side salad for a complete meal.

Leftover drumsticks can be stored in an airtight container in the refrigerator for up to 3 days.

Nutritional Information (per serving, based on 4 servings):

Calories: 300 kcal

Protein: 25g

Carbohydrates: 10g

Fiber: 0g

Fat: 15g

Saturated Fat: 3g

Cholesterol: 120mg

Sodium: 350mg

Potassium: 400mg

These Honey-Garlic Chicken Drumsticks are a flavorful and satisfying dish that fits within the Anti-inflammatory Autoimmune Protocol (AIP) guidelines. The combination of coconut aminos, honey (optional), garlic, and vinegar creates a delicious marinade that caramelizes beautifully on the drumsticks during baking. Enjoy these tender and juicy drumsticks as a comforting and nutritious meal option for any occasion.

Balsamic Glazed Chicken Breasts

Ingredients:
4 chicken breasts, boneless and skinless
1/4 cup balsamic vinegar
2 tablespoons olive oil or avocado oil
2 cloves garlic, minced
1 tablespoon honey (optional, omit for strict AIP)
1 teaspoon dried thyme
Sea salt and freshly ground black pepper, to taste (omit black pepper for strict AIP)
Fresh parsley, chopped (for garnish)

Instructions:
1. In a bowl, whisk together balsamic vinegar, olive oil or avocado oil, minced garlic, honey (if using), dried thyme, sea salt, and freshly ground black pepper (if using).
2. Place chicken breasts in a large resealable plastic bag or shallow dish. Pour the marinade over the chicken breasts, ensuring they are evenly coated. Marinate in the refrigerator for at least 30 minutes, or up to 2 hours for best flavor.
3. Preheat the oven to 400°F (200°C). Line a baking sheet with parchment paper.
4. Remove chicken breasts from the marinade, reserving the marinade for later use.
5. Place chicken breasts on the prepared baking sheet. Bake in the preheated oven for 20-25 minutes, or until chicken is cooked

through and juices run clear, brushing with reserved marinade halfway through cooking.

6. Remove from the oven and let the chicken breasts rest for a few minutes before serving.

7. Garnish with chopped fresh parsley before serving.

Tips/Notes:

Ensure chicken breasts are evenly coated with the marinade for maximum flavor.

Adjust honey quantity based on your sweetness preference or omit entirely for strict AIP.

Serve with roasted vegetables or a side salad for a balanced meal.

Leftover chicken breasts can be stored in an airtight container in the refrigerator for up to 3 days.

Nutritional Information (per serving, based on 4 servings):

Calories: 250 kcal

Protein: 30g

Carbohydrates: 5g

Fiber: 0g

Fat: 10g

Saturated Fat: 2g

Cholesterol: 90mg

Sodium: 300mg

Potassium: 400mg

These Balsamic Glazed Chicken Breasts are a savory and flavorful dish that aligns with the Anti-inflammatory Autoimmune Protocol (AIP) guidelines. The combination of balsamic vinegar, garlic, and herbs creates a delicious glaze that enhances the natural flavor of the chicken breasts. Enjoy this simple yet elegant meal option as a nutritious addition to your AIP-friendly menu.

VI

Sauces and Condiments

Creating flavorful sauces and condiments while adhering to the Anti-inflammatory Autoimmune Protocol (AIP) can be both creative and satisfying. The AIP diet focuses on eliminating potentially inflammatory foods to support gut health and reduce autoimmune symptoms. Thus, sauces and condiments play a crucial role in enhancing dishes without relying on ingredients like dairy, grains, nightshades, or processed sugars.

AIP-friendly sauces and condiments often use ingredients such as coconut aminos as a soy sauce substitute, apple cider vinegar for tanginess, and various herbs and spices for flavor. These ingredients not only add depth but also align with the dietary restrictions of the AIP protocol. Examples of AIP sauces include creamy coconut milk-based dressings, citrus-infused vinaigrettes, and herbaceous pestos made with compliant ingredients.

Experimenting with homemade AIP sauces allows for customization to personal taste preferences while ensuring all components are supportive of the diet's principles. By focusing on natural ingredients and avoiding additives, individuals on the AIP diet can enjoy flavorful meals without compromising their health goals. Whether drizzling over proteins, dressing salads, or dipping vegetables, AIP sauces and condiments can elevate any dish while promoting wellness and inflammation reduction.

AIP-Friendly Ketchup

Ingredients:
1 cup unsweetened applesauce
1/4 cup apple cider vinegar
1 tablespoon honey (optional, omit for strict AIP)
1 teaspoon garlic powder
1 teaspoon onion powder
1/2 teaspoon sea salt

Instructions:
1. In a saucepan, combine unsweetened applesauce, apple cider vinegar, honey (if using), garlic powder, onion powder, and sea salt.
2. Stir well to combine all ingredients.
3. Bring the mixture to a simmer over medium heat.
4. Reduce heat to low and let it simmer gently for 20-25 minutes, stirring occasionally, until the ketchup thickens to your desired consistency.
5. Remove from heat and let it cool completely.
6. Transfer the ketchup to a sealed container or jar and refrigerate.

Tips/Notes:
Adjust sweetness and tanginess by varying the amount of honey and apple cider vinegar to suit your taste.

Store the AIP-friendly ketchup in the refrigerator for up to 2 weeks.
Use this ketchup as a dipping sauce or condiment for AIP-compliant dishes like sweet potato fries, burgers, or meatloaf.

Nutritional Information (per serving, based on approximately 2 tablespoons):
Calories: 20 kcal
Carbohydrates: 5g
Fiber: 1g
Sugars: 4g
Fat: 0g
Protein: 0g
Sodium: 100mg

Creamy Avocado Dressing

Ingredients:
1 ripe avocado, peeled and pitted
1/4 cup coconut milk (full-fat)
2 tablespoons fresh lemon juice
1 tablespoon extra virgin olive oil
1 clove garlic, minced
Sea salt and freshly ground black pepper, to taste (omit black pepper for strict AIP)

Instructions:
1. In a blender or food processor, combine the ripe avocado, coconut milk, fresh lemon juice, extra virgin olive oil, minced garlic, sea salt, and freshly ground black pepper (if using).

2. Blend until smooth and creamy, scraping down the sides as needed to ensure all ingredients are well combined.
3. Taste and adjust seasoning, adding more salt or lemon juice as desired.
4. If the dressing is too thick, you can thin it out with a little more coconut milk or water.
5. Transfer the creamy avocado dressing to a sealed container or jar.
6. Refrigerate for at least 30 minutes to allow the flavors to meld before serving.

Tips/Notes:
Use this creamy avocado dressing as a salad dressing, dip for vegetables, or sauce for grilled chicken or fish.
Store leftovers in an airtight container in the refrigerator for up to 3 days.
For a variation, you can add fresh herbs like cilantro or parsley for added flavor.

Nutritional Information (per serving, based on approximately 2 tablespoons):
Calories: 60 kcal
Carbohydrates: 3g
Fiber: 2g
Sugars: 0g
Fat: 5g
Saturated Fat: 2g
Protein: 1g
Sodium: 50mg

This Creamy Avocado Dressing is a delicious and nutritious option that aligns with the Anti-inflammatory Autoimmune Protocol (AIP) guidelines. It utilizes avocado for creaminess, coconut milk for richness, and fresh lemon juice for tanginess, creating a versatile dressing or dip that enhances AIP-friendly meals.

Coconut Amino Teriyaki Sauce

Ingredients:
1/2 cup coconut aminos
1/4 cup water
2 tablespoons honey (optional, omit for strict AIP)
1 tablespoon apple cider vinegar
1 clove garlic, minced
1 teaspoon fresh ginger, grated
1 tablespoon arrowroot powder (or tapioca starch), dissolved in 2 tablespoons water

Instructions:
1. In a small saucepan, combine coconut aminos, water, honey (if using), apple cider vinegar, minced garlic, and grated ginger.
2. Bring the mixture to a simmer over medium heat, stirring occasionally.
3. Once simmering, slowly pour in the arrowroot powder (or tapioca starch) mixture while stirring continuously to prevent clumping.
4. Cook the sauce for 3-5 minutes, or until it thickens to your desired consistency.
5. Remove from heat and let it cool slightly before using.

Tips/Notes:
Adjust sweetness and saltiness by varying the amount of honey and coconut aminos.

Use this teriyaki sauce as a marinade for meats or vegetables, or as a sauce for stir-fries and rice dishes.

Store any leftover sauce in a sealed container in the refrigerator for up to 1 week.

For a richer flavor, you can add a dash of sesame oil (if tolerated) or substitute some of the water with pineapple juice.

Nutritional Information (per serving, based on approximately 2 tablespoons):
Calories: 30 kcal
Carbohydrates: 7g
Fiber: 0g
Sugars: 5g
Fat: 0g
Protein: 0g
Sodium: 300mg

This Coconut Amino Teriyaki Sauce is a flavorful and versatile option that complies with the Anti-inflammatory Autoimmune Protocol (AIP) guidelines. It offers a balance of savory, sweet, and tangy flavors, making it ideal for enhancing a variety of AIP-friendly dishes while avoiding common inflammatory ingredients.

Garlic Aioli

Ingredients:
1/2 cup coconut cream (from a refrigerated can of coconut milk)
2 cloves garlic, minced
2 tablespoons extra virgin olive oil
1 tablespoon fresh lemon juice

Sea salt, to taste
Fresh parsley, chopped (optional, for garnish)

Instructions:
1. Scoop out the thick coconut cream from a refrigerated can of coconut milk, leaving the watery part behind.
2. In a small bowl, combine the coconut cream, minced garlic, extra virgin olive oil, fresh lemon juice, and a pinch of sea salt.
3. Use a whisk or immersion blender to blend the ingredients until smooth and creamy.
4. Taste and adjust seasoning, adding more salt or lemon juice as needed.
5. If the aioli is too thick, you can thin it out with a little water or more lemon juice.
6. Transfer the garlic aioli to a serving bowl and garnish with chopped fresh parsley, if desired.

Tips/Notes:
Use this garlic aioli as a dip for vegetables, a spread for burgers or sandwiches, or a sauce for grilled chicken or fish.
Store leftovers in an airtight container in the refrigerator for up to 3 days.
For a variation, you can add chopped herbs like chives or basil for added flavor.

Nutritional Information (per serving, based on approximately 2 tablespoons):
Calories: 80 kcal
Carbohydrates: 2g
Fiber: 0g
Sugars: 0g
Fat: 8g
Saturated Fat: 5g

Protein: 0g
Sodium: 50mg

This Garlic Aioli is a creamy and dairy-free alternative that aligns with the Anti-inflammatory Autoimmune Protocol (AIP) guidelines. It uses coconut cream for richness, garlic for flavor, and olive oil for smoothness, creating a versatile condiment that enhances AIP-friendly meals. Enjoy this flavorful aioli as a delicious addition to your favorite dishes without compromising on dietary restrictions.

Herb-Infused Olive Oil

Creating herb-infused olive oil is a simple process that adds depth and flavor to dishes while adhering to the Anti-inflammatory Autoimmune Protocol (AIP). Here's a basic outline to guide you through making Herb-Infused Olive Oil:

Ingredients:
1 cup extra virgin olive oil
Fresh herbs of your choice (e.g., rosemary, thyme, oregano, basil), washed and dried

Instructions:
1. Wash and thoroughly dry the fresh herbs to remove any moisture.
2. Bruise or lightly crush the herbs with a mortar and pestle or by gently rubbing them between your hands to release their flavors.
3. In a small saucepan, heat the olive oil over low heat until it reaches about 180°F (82°C).
4. Place the dried herbs into a clean glass jar or bottle.

5. Carefully pour the warm olive oil over the herbs, ensuring they are completely submerged.

6. Seal the jar or bottle tightly with a lid.

7. Let the herb-infused olive oil cool to room temperature, then store it in a cool, dark place for at least 1 week to allow the flavors to develop.

8. Strain the oil through a fine-mesh sieve or cheesecloth into a clean container to remove the herbs.

9. Seal the infused olive oil and store it in the refrigerator for up to 1 month.

Tips/Notes:

Use herb-infused olive oil as a dressing for salads, a drizzle over roasted vegetables, or as a marinade for meats.

Experiment with different combinations of herbs to customize the flavor to your preference.

Ensure all utensils and containers used are clean and dry to prevent spoilage.

Discard any infused oil that shows signs of cloudiness, mold, or an off odor.

Nutritional Information (per tablespoon):

Calories: 120 kcal

Fat: 14g

Saturated Fat: 2g

Polyunsaturated Fat: 1.5g

Monounsaturated Fat: 10g

Sodium: 0mg

Carbohydrates: 0g

Fiber: 0g

Sugars: 0g

Protein: 0g

Enjoy this Herb-Infused Olive Oil as a flavorful and versatile addition to your AIP-friendly kitchen, enhancing dishes with the natural essence of fresh herbs and the health benefits of high-quality olive oil.

Lemon Tahini Sauce

Ingredients:
1/2 cup tahini (sesame seed paste)
1/4 cup water
2 tablespoons fresh lemon juice
1 clove garlic, minced
1 tablespoon extra virgin olive oil
Sea salt, to taste

Instructions:
1. In a small bowl or food processor, combine tahini, water, fresh lemon juice, minced garlic, extra virgin olive oil, and a pinch of sea salt.
2. Blend or whisk until smooth and creamy, adjusting consistency with more water if needed.
3. Taste and adjust seasoning, adding more salt or lemon juice as desired.
4. Transfer the lemon tahini sauce to a serving bowl.

Tips/Notes:
Use this lemon tahini sauce as a dressing for salads, a dip for vegetables, or a sauce for grilled meats or fish.
Store leftover sauce in an airtight container in the refrigerator for up to 5 days.

For added flavor, you can mix in chopped herbs like parsley or cilantro.

Adjust the thickness by adding more water for a thinner consistency or reducing water for a thicker sauce.

Nutritional Information (per serving, based on approximately 2 tablespoons):
Calories: 100 kcal
Fat: 9g
Saturated Fat: 1g
Sodium: 50mg
Carbohydrates: 4g
Fiber: 1g
Sugars: 0g
Protein: 3g

This Lemon Tahini Sauce is a creamy and tangy condiment that complements a variety of dishes while adhering to the Anti-inflammatory Autoimmune Protocol (AIP) guidelines. Enjoy its rich flavor and versatility in enhancing AIP-friendly meals.

AIP BBQ Sauce

Ingredients:
1 cup unsweetened applesauce
1/4 cup apple cider vinegar
2 tablespoons coconut aminos
1 tablespoon honey (optional, omit for strict AIP)
1 teaspoon garlic powder
1 teaspoon onion powder

1/2 teaspoon ground ginger
Sea salt, to taste

Instructions:
1. In a saucepan, combine unsweetened applesauce, apple cider vinegar, coconut aminos, honey (if using), garlic powder, onion powder, ground ginger, and a pinch of sea salt.
2. Stir well to combine all ingredients.
3. Bring the mixture to a simmer over medium heat, stirring occasionally.
4. Reduce heat to low and let it simmer gently for 15-20 minutes, stirring occasionally, until the sauce thickens.
5. Taste and adjust seasoning, adding more salt or honey (if desired) to achieve your preferred taste.
6. Remove from heat and let it cool slightly before using.

Tips/Notes:
Use this AIP BBQ sauce as a marinade for meats, a glaze for grilled vegetables, or a dipping sauce for AIP-friendly nuggets or wings.
Store any leftover sauce in a sealed container in the refrigerator for up to 1 week.
For a smokier flavor, you can add a small amount of smoked paprika (if tolerated) or use smoked salt.
Adjust sweetness and tanginess by varying the amount of honey and apple cider vinegar according to your taste preferences.

Nutritional Information (per serving, based on approximately 2 tablespoons):
Calories: 30 kcal
Carbohydrates: 7g
Fiber: 1g
Sugars: 5g
Fat: 0g

Protein: 0g
Sodium: 100mg

This AIP BBQ Sauce provides a sweet, tangy flavor profile that aligns with the Anti-inflammatory Autoimmune Protocol (AIP) guidelines, making it suitable for those managing autoimmune conditions. Enjoy this sauce to enhance the flavor of your favorite AIP meals while avoiding common inflammatory ingredients.

Ginger Carrot Dressing

Ingredients:
1 large carrot, peeled and chopped
1-inch piece of fresh ginger, peeled and chopped
2 tablespoons rice vinegar (or apple cider vinegar for AIP)
1 tablespoon coconut aminos
1 tablespoon extra virgin olive oil
1 tablespoon water
1 teaspoon honey (optional, omit for strict AIP)
Sea salt, to taste

Instructions:
1. In a blender or food processor, combine chopped carrot, fresh ginger, rice vinegar (or apple cider vinegar), coconut aminos, extra virgin olive oil, water, honey (if using), and a pinch of sea salt.
2. Blend until smooth and creamy, scraping down the sides as needed to ensure all ingredients are well combined.
3. Taste and adjust seasoning, adding more salt or honey (if desired) to suit your taste preferences.

4. If the dressing is too thick, you can thin it out with a little more water or vinegar.

5. Transfer the ginger carrot dressing to a serving bowl or container.

Tips/Notes:

Use this ginger carrot dressing as a salad dressing, a sauce for grain bowls, or a marinade for chicken or tofu.

Store any leftover dressing in a sealed container in the refrigerator for up to 3-4 days.

For added flavor, you can add a splash of sesame oil (if tolerated) or a sprinkle of sesame seeds before serving.

Adjust the ginger amount according to your preference for a stronger or milder ginger flavor.

Nutritional Information (per serving, based on approximately 2 tablespoons):

Calories: 40 kcal

Carbohydrates: 5g

Fiber: 1g

Sugars: 3g

Fat: 2g

Saturated Fat: 0g

Protein: 0g

Sodium: 100mg

This Ginger Carrot Dressing offers a refreshing and tangy addition to salads and meals, suitable for those following the Anti-inflammatory Autoimmune Protocol (AIP) guidelines. Enjoy its vibrant flavors while supporting your dietary preferences and health goals.

I'm currently unable to provide specific recipes. However, here's a general outline you can use to create your Cilantro Lime Dressing:

Cilantro Lime Dressing

Ingredients:
1 cup fresh cilantro leaves, packed
Juice and zest of 1 lime
1/4 cup extra virgin olive oil
1 tablespoon apple cider vinegar (or coconut vinegar for AIP)
1 clove garlic, minced
Sea salt, to taste

Instructions:
1. In a blender or food processor, combine fresh cilantro leaves, lime juice and zest, extra virgin olive oil, apple cider vinegar (or coconut vinegar), minced garlic, and a pinch of sea salt.
2. Blend until smooth and well combined, scraping down the sides as needed.
3. Taste and adjust seasoning, adding more salt or lime juice to suit your taste preferences.
4. If the dressing is too thick, you can thin it out with a little water or more olive oil.
5. Transfer the cilantro lime dressing to a serving bowl or container.

Tips/Notes:
Use this cilantro lime dressing as a topping for salads, a marinade for grilled chicken or seafood, or a dipping sauce for vegetables.

Store any leftover dressing in a sealed container in the refrigerator for up to 3-4 days.

For added heat, you can add a pinch of red pepper flakes or a dash of hot sauce.

Adjust the amount of cilantro and lime juice according to your preference for a stronger or milder flavor.

Nutritional Information (per serving, based on approximately 2 tablespoons):
Calories: 80 kcal
Carbohydrates: 1g
Fiber: 0g
Sugars: 0g
Fat: 9g
Saturated Fat: 1g
Protein: 0g
Sodium: 50mg

This Cilantro Lime Dressing offers a zesty and herbaceous flavor profile, perfect for enhancing salads and dishes while adhering to the Anti-inflammatory Autoimmune Protocol (AIP) guidelines. Enjoy its fresh taste and versatility in your AIP-friendly meals.

Nut-Free Basil Pesto

Ingredients:
2 cups fresh basil leaves, packed
1/4 cup extra virgin olive oil
2 cloves garlic, minced
2 tablespoons nutritional yeast

Juice of 1 lemon
Sea salt, to taste

Instructions:
1. In a food processor or blender, combine fresh basil leaves, extra virgin olive oil, minced garlic, nutritional yeast, lemon juice, and a pinch of sea salt.
2. Pulse or blend until the mixture becomes a smooth paste, scraping down the sides as needed.
3. Taste and adjust seasoning, adding more salt or lemon juice to suit your taste preferences.
4. If the pesto is too thick, you can add a little more olive oil to achieve your desired consistency.
5. Transfer the nut-free basil pesto to a serving bowl or container.

Tips/Notes:
Use this nut-free basil pesto as a sauce for pasta, a spread for sandwiches or wraps, or a topping for grilled vegetables.
Store any leftover pesto in a sealed container in the refrigerator for up to 3-4 days.
For a variation, you can add a handful of fresh spinach or kale for added nutrition and flavor.
Adjust the garlic amount according to your preference for a stronger or milder garlic flavor.

Nutritional Information (per serving, based on approximately 2 tablespoons):
Calories: 80 kcal
Carbohydrates: 2g
Fiber: 1g
Sugars: 0g
Fat: 8g
Saturated Fat: 1g

Protein: 1g
Sodium: 50mg

This Nut-Free Basil Pesto offers a vibrant and herbaceous flavor profile, perfect for those following a nut-free diet or the Anti-inflammatory Autoimmune Protocol (AIP) guidelines. Enjoy its versatility and fresh taste in a variety of AIP-friendly dishes.

Coconut Milk Ranch Dressing

Ingredients:
1/2 cup full-fat coconut milk (from a can)
1/4 cup coconut cream (from the top of a refrigerated can of coconut milk)
1 tablespoon apple cider vinegar (or lemon juice for AIP)
1 clove garlic, minced
1/2 teaspoon onion powder
1/2 teaspoon dried dill
1/2 teaspoon dried parsley
Sea salt, to taste

Instructions:
1. In a mixing bowl, combine full-fat coconut milk, coconut cream, apple cider vinegar (or lemon juice), minced garlic, onion powder, dried dill, dried parsley, and a pinch of sea salt.
2. Whisk all ingredients together until smooth and well combined.
3. Taste and adjust seasoning, adding more salt or herbs to suit your taste preferences.
4. For a thicker consistency, refrigerate the dressing for about 30 minutes before serving.

5. Transfer the coconut milk ranch dressing to a serving bowl or container.

Tips/Notes:
Use this coconut milk ranch dressing as a dip for vegetables, a dressing for salads, or a sauce for AIP-friendly chicken tenders or wraps.
Store any leftover dressing in a sealed container in the refrigerator for up to 3-4 days.
For added flavor, you can add a dash of smoked paprika or a squeeze of fresh lemon juice.
Adjust the thickness by adding more coconut cream or coconut milk as needed.

Nutritional Information (per serving, based on approximately 2 tablespoons):
Calories: 80 kcal
Carbohydrates: 2g
Fiber: 0g
Sugars: 0g
Fat: 8g
Saturated Fat: 7g
Protein: 1g
Sodium: 50mg

This Coconut Milk Ranch Dressing offers a creamy and dairy-free alternative to traditional ranch dressing, suitable for those following the Anti-inflammatory Autoimmune Protocol (AIP) guidelines. Enjoy its rich flavor and versatility in enhancing AIP-friendly meals.

Roasted Red Pepper Dip

Ingredients:
2 large red bell peppers
1/4 cup tahini (sesame seed paste)
2 tablespoons extra virgin olive oil
1 clove garlic, minced
Juice of 1 lemon
Sea salt, to taste

Instructions:
1. Preheat the oven to 400°F (200°C). Line a baking sheet with parchment paper.
2. Place the whole red bell peppers on the baking sheet and roast in the preheated oven for 30-40 minutes, turning occasionally, until the peppers are charred and softened.
3. Remove the peppers from the oven and let them cool slightly. Once cool enough to handle, peel off the charred skin, remove the seeds, and roughly chop the roasted peppers.
4. In a food processor or blender, combine the roasted red peppers, tahini, extra virgin olive oil, minced garlic, lemon juice, and a pinch of sea salt.
5. Blend until smooth and creamy, scraping down the sides as needed to ensure all ingredients are well combined.
6. Taste and adjust seasoning, adding more salt or lemon juice to suit your taste preferences.
7. Transfer the roasted red pepper dip to a serving bowl.

Tips/Notes:

Serve this roasted red pepper dip with raw vegetable sticks, gluten-free crackers, or as a spread on sandwiches or wraps.
Store any leftover dip in a sealed container in the refrigerator for up to 3-4 days.
For a smokier flavor, you can add a dash of smoked paprika or a pinch of cumin.
Adjust the garlic amount according to your preference for a stronger or milder garlic flavor.

Nutritional Information (per serving, based on approximately 2 tablespoons):
Calories: 60 kcal
Carbohydrates: 3g
Fiber: 1g
Sugars: 1g
Fat: 5g
Saturated Fat: 1g
Protein: 1g
Sodium: 100mg

This Roasted Red Pepper Dip offers a savory and smoky flavor profile, perfect for dipping and spreading while adhering to the Anti-inflammatory Autoimmune Protocol (AIP) guidelines. Enjoy its versatility and robust taste in your AIP-friendly meals and snacks.

VII

Drinks and Teas

Drinks and teas play a crucial role in the Anti-inflammatory Autoimmune Protocol (AIP), providing hydration and potential therapeutic benefits. In this protocol, beverages are chosen not only for their taste but also for their ability to support gut health, reduce inflammation, and avoid common triggers that may exacerbate autoimmune conditions.

AIP-compliant drinks typically exclude alcohol, caffeine, and processed sugars. Instead, they often feature herbal teas, bone broths, and nutrient-dense beverages like homemade nut milks or coconut water. These choices are designed to be soothing to the digestive system while providing essential vitamins and minerals.

Herbal teas are particularly favored in AIP for their calming properties and potential anti-inflammatory effects. Teas such as chamomile, ginger, and peppermint are popular choices, known for their digestive support and stress-relieving benefits. Bone broth, rich in collagen and amino acids, is another staple, believed to support gut integrity and overall immune function.

Innovative AIP recipes also explore homemade nut milks, infused waters, and herbal tonics that harness the healing power of ingredients like turmeric, ginger, and medicinal herbs. By focusing on these nourishing beverages, individuals following the AIP can enhance their overall well-being and manage autoimmune symptoms effectively.

Turmeric Golden Milk

Ingredients:
1 cup unsweetened coconut milk (or almond milk for AIP)
1 teaspoon ground turmeric
1/2 teaspoon ground cinnamon
1/4 teaspoon ground ginger
Pinch of ground black pepper
1 teaspoon raw honey (optional, omit for strict AIP)
1/2 teaspoon coconut oil
1/2 teaspoon vanilla extract (optional)

Instructions:
1. In a small saucepan, heat the unsweetened coconut milk (or almond milk) over medium heat until warmed but not boiling.
2. Whisk in ground turmeric, ground cinnamon, ground ginger, a pinch of ground black pepper, raw honey (if using), coconut oil, and vanilla extract (if using).
3. Continue to whisk gently until all ingredients are well combined and the mixture is heated through.
4. Taste and adjust sweetness or spices according to your preference.

5. Remove from heat and pour the turmeric golden milk into a mug.

Tips/Notes:
Turmeric golden milk can be enjoyed hot or cold.
Stir the mixture occasionally while heating to ensure the spices are well blended.
Customize the sweetness by adjusting the amount of honey or using alternative sweeteners like maple syrup or stevia.
Turmeric has natural staining properties, so be cautious to avoid spills on clothing or countertops.

Nutritional Information (per serving, based on approximately 1 cup):
Calories: 70 kcal
Carbohydrates: 4g
Fiber: 1g
Sugars: 2g
Fat: 5g
Saturated Fat: 4g
Protein: 1g
Sodium: 10mg

This Turmeric Golden Milk offers a comforting and anti-inflammatory beverage option, perfect for those following the Anti-inflammatory Autoimmune Protocol (AIP). Enjoy its soothing qualities and potential health benefits as part of your daily routine.

Mint and Ginger Iced Tea

Ingredients:
4 cups water
1/4 cup fresh mint leaves
1-inch piece of fresh ginger, thinly sliced
Juice of 1 lemon
Honey or maple syrup to taste (optional, omit for strict AIP)
Ice cubes

Instructions:
1. In a medium saucepan, bring 4 cups of water to a boil.
2. Remove the saucepan from heat and add fresh mint leaves and thinly sliced ginger.
3. Cover the saucepan and let the mixture steep for about 10-15 minutes.
4. Strain the mint and ginger from the tea, discarding the solids.
5. Allow the tea to cool to room temperature, then refrigerate until chilled.
6. Once chilled, stir in the juice of 1 lemon and sweeten with honey or maple syrup if desired.
7. Fill glasses with ice cubes and pour the mint and ginger iced tea over the ice.
8. Garnish with additional mint leaves or lemon slices if desired.

Tips/Notes:
Adjust the steeping time for a stronger or milder flavor.
For a stronger ginger taste, grate the ginger instead of slicing it.
You can make a larger batch and store it in the refrigerator for up to 2-3 days.

Experiment with different sweeteners or herbal additions like chamomile for variety.

Nutritional Information (per serving, based on approximately 1 cup):
Calories: 10 kcal
Carbohydrates: 3g
Fiber: 0g
Sugars: 1g
Fat: 0g
Protein: 0g
Sodium: 0mg

This Mint and Ginger Iced Tea offers a refreshing and hydrating beverage option, suitable for those following the Anti-inflammatory Autoimmune Protocol (AIP). Enjoy its crisp flavors and potential health benefits on warm days or as a cooling treat.

Cucumber Basil Water

Ingredients:
1 cucumber, thinly sliced
1/4 cup fresh basil leaves
4 cups water
Ice cubes

Instructions:
1. In a large pitcher, combine thinly sliced cucumber and fresh basil leaves.
2. Pour 4 cups of water over the cucumber and basil.
3. Stir gently to mix the ingredients.
4. Cover the pitcher and refrigerate for at least 2 hours to allow the flavors to infuse.

5. Serve the cucumber basil water over ice cubes.

Tips/Notes:
For a stronger flavor, muddle the basil leaves slightly before adding them to the pitcher.
You can adjust the amount of cucumber and basil according to your taste preferences.
This infused water can be stored in the refrigerator for up to 2 days.
Customize by adding other herbs like mint or lemon slices for variation.

Nutritional Information:
Since this is primarily infused water, the nutritional information can vary widely based on personal consumption and how long the ingredients are infused. Generally, infused water is low in calories and carbohydrates, making it a refreshing and hydrating option without added sugars or artificial ingredients.

Anti-inflammatory Smoothie

Ingredients:
1 cup unsweetened almond milk (or coconut milk for AIP)
1/2 cup frozen berries (such as blueberries, strawberries, or raspberries)
1/2 inch piece of fresh ginger, peeled and grated
1/2 teaspoon ground turmeric
1 tablespoon chia seeds
1 tablespoon collagen powder (optional)
Ice cubes (optional)

Instructions:
1. In a blender, combine unsweetened almond milk (or coconut milk), frozen berries, grated fresh ginger, ground turmeric, chia seeds, and collagen powder (if using).
2. Blend on high speed until smooth and well combined, adding ice cubes if a colder consistency is desired.
3. Taste and adjust sweetness or spice levels as needed by adding a small amount of honey, maple syrup, or a few drops of stevia (optional).
4. Pour the smoothie into a glass and serve immediately.

Tips/Notes:
Adjust the thickness of the smoothie by adding more or less almond milk/coconut milk.
To enhance the flavor and nutrition, consider adding a handful of spinach or kale leaves.
For extra creaminess, include half an avocado or a scoop of coconut yogurt.
Experiment with different berries or add a squeeze of lemon juice for variation.

Nutritional Information (per serving, based on approximately 1 cup):
Calories: 150 kcal
Carbohydrates: 15g
Fiber: 7g
Sugars: 5g
Fat: 7g
Saturated Fat: 1g
Protein: 7g
Sodium: 100mg

This Anti-inflammatory Smoothie is packed with antioxidants, anti-inflammatory ingredients, and nutrients, making it an excellent choice for those following the Anti-inflammatory Autoimmune Protocol (AIP). Enjoy its refreshing taste and potential health benefits as part of your balanced diet.

Herbal Chai Tea

Ingredients:
4 cups water
1 cinnamon stick
4-6 whole cloves
4-6 whole cardamom pods
1-inch piece of fresh ginger, sliced
1 star anise (optional)
1/4 teaspoon ground nutmeg
1/4 teaspoon ground black pepper
1/4 teaspoon ground fennel seeds
Honey or maple syrup to taste (optional, omit for strict AIP)
Unsweetened coconut milk or almond milk (optional)

Instructions:
1. In a medium saucepan, bring 4 cups of water to a boil.
2. Add the cinnamon stick, whole cloves, whole cardamom pods, sliced fresh ginger, star anise (if using), ground nutmeg, ground black pepper, and ground fennel seeds to the boiling water.
3. Reduce the heat to low and simmer the mixture for about 10-15 minutes to allow the flavors to meld.
4. Remove the saucepan from heat and let the chai tea steep for an additional 5 minutes.

5. Strain the herbal chai tea into a teapot or serving pitcher, discarding the spices and ginger.

6. Sweeten the chai tea with honey or maple syrup if desired.

7. Serve the herbal chai tea hot, optionally with unsweetened coconut milk or almond milk.

Tips/Notes:

Adjust the spice levels according to your taste preferences.

For a stronger flavor, steep the tea for a longer period before straining.

Use organic ingredients whenever possible to ensure purity and quality.

Store any leftover chai tea in a sealed container in the refrigerator for up to 2 days.

Nutritional Information:

Herbal chai tea is primarily water-based and low in calories. The nutritional content varies based on the specific ingredients and optional additions like honey or milk. Enjoy this warming and aromatic beverage as a comforting treat, suitable for those following the Anti-inflammatory Autoimmune Protocol (AIP).

Coconut Matcha Latte

Ingredients:

1 teaspoon matcha powder

1 cup hot water (not boiling, around 175°F or 80°C)

1/2 cup unsweetened coconut milk

1 teaspoon raw honey or maple syrup (optional, omit for strict AIP)

Optional: 1/4 teaspoon vanilla extract

Instructions:
1. In a small bowl or matcha bowl, sift the matcha powder to remove any clumps.
2. Add hot water (not boiling) to the matcha powder.
3. Use a bamboo whisk or a small whisk to vigorously whisk the matcha and water together until frothy and well combined.
4. In a small saucepan, heat the unsweetened coconut milk over medium heat until warmed, but not boiling.
5. Remove from heat and whisk in raw honey or maple syrup (if using) and vanilla extract (if using).
6. Pour the warmed coconut milk into a mug.
7. Slowly pour the prepared matcha mixture over the coconut milk, using a spoon to hold back the froth if desired.
8. Stir gently to combine, ensuring the matcha is evenly distributed.
9. Optionally, garnish with a sprinkle of matcha powder on top for presentation.

Tips/Notes:
Adjust the sweetness by adding more or less honey/maple syrup.
Ensure the water used for matcha is not boiling to prevent bitterness.
For a creamier texture, use full-fat coconut milk or add a splash of coconut cream.
Experiment with different types of sweeteners or alternative milks like almond or cashew milk.

Nutritional Information:
Matcha is rich in antioxidants and provides a moderate amount of caffeine, making this latte a refreshing and energizing choice. The nutritional content can vary based on specific ingredients and optional additions. Enjoy this Coconut Matcha Latte as a

nourishing beverage suitable for those following the Anti-inflammatory Autoimmune Protocol (AIP).

Lavender Lemonade

Ingredients:
4 cups water
1/4 cup dried culinary lavender buds
1 cup freshly squeezed lemon juice (about 4-6 lemons)
1/2 cup raw honey or maple syrup (adjust to taste, omit for strict AIP)
Ice cubes
Lemon slices and fresh lavender sprigs for garnish (optional)

Instructions:
1. In a medium saucepan, bring 4 cups of water to a boil.
2. Remove the saucepan from heat and add dried culinary lavender buds.
3. Cover the saucepan and let the lavender steep in the hot water for about 20-30 minutes.
4. Strain the lavender-infused water through a fine mesh sieve or cheesecloth into a large pitcher, discarding the lavender buds.
5. Stir in freshly squeezed lemon juice and raw honey or maple syrup (if using), adjusting sweetness to taste.
6. Chill the lavender lemonade in the refrigerator for at least 1 hour or until cold.
7. Serve the lavender lemonade over ice cubes in glasses.
8. Garnish with lemon slices and fresh lavender sprigs if desired.

Tips/Notes:

Adjust the amount of honey or maple syrup based on your preference for sweetness.

For a stronger lavender flavor, steep the buds longer or use more lavender buds.

Store any leftover lavender lemonade in the refrigerator for up to 2 days.

Use organic ingredients whenever possible to ensure purity.

Nutritional Information:

Lavender lemonade is primarily water-based and low in calories. The nutritional content can vary based on the specific ingredients and optional additions like honey or maple syrup. Enjoy this floral and refreshing beverage as a delightful treat, suitable for those following the Anti-inflammatory Autoimmune Protocol (AIP).

Beet and Berry Smoothie

Ingredients:

1 small beet, peeled and chopped (or use pre-cooked beet for easier blending)

1 cup mixed berries (such as strawberries, blueberries, raspberries)

1 banana, peeled and sliced (omit for strict AIP)

1 cup unsweetened almond milk (or coconut milk for AIP)

1 tablespoon chia seeds

Ice cubes (optional)

Instructions:

1. In a blender, combine chopped beet, mixed berries, banana (if using), unsweetened almond milk, and chia seeds.

2. Blend on high speed until smooth and creamy. Add ice cubes if desired for a colder smoothie.

3. Taste and adjust sweetness or texture by adding a small amount of honey or maple syrup (optional).

4. Blend again until well combined and smooth.

5. Pour the beet and berry smoothie into glasses and serve immediately.

Tips/Notes:
Adjust the thickness of the smoothie by adding more or less almond milk/coconut milk.
For added nutrition, consider adding a handful of spinach or kale leaves.
Chia seeds provide additional fiber and omega-3 fatty acids.
Customize with other fruits like mango or pineapple for variety.

Nutritional Information:
Since this is primarily fruit and vegetable-based, the nutritional content will vary based on the specific ingredients used. Generally, this smoothie is low in calories and rich in vitamins, minerals, and antioxidants, making it a nutritious choice suitable for those following the Anti-inflammatory Autoimmune Protocol (AIP).

AIP Hot Chocolate

Ingredients:
1 cup unsweetened coconut milk or almond milk (check for compliance with AIP)
2 tablespoons carob powder (AIP-friendly alternative to cocoa powder)
1/2 teaspoon ground cinnamon
1/4 teaspoon ground ginger

1/8 teaspoon ground cloves

1/8 teaspoon ground nutmeg (omit for strict AIP)

1 tablespoon raw honey or maple syrup (adjust to taste, omit for strict AIP)

Optional: 1/4 teaspoon vanilla extract (omit for strict AIP)

Instructions:

1. In a small saucepan, heat unsweetened coconut milk or almond milk over medium heat until warmed but not boiling.

2. Whisk in carob powder, ground cinnamon, ground ginger, ground cloves, and ground nutmeg (if using).

3. Continue whisking until the mixture is smooth and well combined.

4. Stir in raw honey or maple syrup (if using) and vanilla extract (if using), adjusting sweetness to taste.

5. Heat the hot chocolate mixture until it reaches your desired temperature.

6. Pour the AIP hot chocolate into mugs and serve immediately.

Tips/Notes:

Adjust the spices according to your preference for a stronger or milder flavor.

Use carob powder instead of cocoa powder to adhere to AIP guidelines.

For a creamier texture, add a splash of coconut cream or full-fat coconut milk.

Top with coconut whipped cream (if tolerated) or a sprinkle of cinnamon for extra flavor.

Nutritional Information:

Since this hot chocolate is primarily plant-based and free from dairy and refined sugars, it tends to be lower in calories and can be a comforting treat for those following the Anti-inflammatory

Autoimmune Protocol (AIP). Adjust ingredients and sweetness levels as needed to suit your dietary preferences.

Lemon Ginger Detox Tea

Ingredients:
4 cups water
1 lemon, sliced
1-inch piece of fresh ginger, sliced
Optional: 1 tablespoon raw honey or maple syrup (omit for strict AIP)

Instructions:
1. In a medium saucepan, bring 4 cups of water to a boil.
2. Add sliced lemon and fresh ginger to the boiling water.
3. Reduce the heat to low and simmer the mixture for about 10-15 minutes to infuse the flavors.
4. Remove the saucepan from heat and let the lemon ginger tea steep for an additional 5 minutes.
5. Strain the tea through a fine mesh sieve or cheesecloth into a teapot or serving pitcher, discarding the lemon slices and ginger.
6. Stir in raw honey or maple syrup if using, adjusting sweetness to taste.
7. Serve the lemon ginger detox tea hot.

Tips/Notes:
Adjust the intensity of ginger by adding more or less slices.
For a stronger lemon flavor, add more lemon slices or squeeze lemon juice directly into the tea.

Enjoy this tea as a refreshing beverage throughout the day to promote hydration and detoxification.
Store any leftover tea in the refrigerator and reheat gently before serving.

Nutritional Information:
This lemon ginger detox tea is naturally low in calories and sugar, making it a healthy and hydrating choice. The nutritional content may vary based on the amount of honey or maple syrup added. It's suitable for those following the Anti-inflammatory Autoimmune Protocol (AIP) and can be enjoyed as part of a balanced diet.

Cinnamon Apple Cider

Ingredients:
4 cups apple juice or apple cider (look for varieties without added sugar)
2 cinnamon sticks
4-6 whole cloves
1/4 teaspoon ground nutmeg
Optional: 1-2 tablespoons raw honey or maple syrup (omit for strict AIP)

Instructions:
1. In a medium saucepan, combine apple juice or apple cider with cinnamon sticks, whole cloves, and ground nutmeg.
2. Bring the mixture to a simmer over medium heat.
3. Reduce the heat to low and let the cider simmer for about 15-20 minutes to infuse the flavors.

4. Remove the saucepan from heat and discard the cinnamon sticks and whole cloves.

5. Stir in raw honey or maple syrup if using, adjusting sweetness to taste.

6. Serve the cinnamon apple cider warm in mugs.

Tips/Notes:

For a stronger cinnamon flavor, break the cinnamon sticks before adding to the cider.

Adjust the sweetness by adding more or less honey or maple syrup.

Garnish with a cinnamon stick or a sprinkle of ground cinnamon for presentation.

This drink can be enjoyed as a comforting beverage during cooler weather or as a festive treat.

Nutritional Information:

This cinnamon apple cider is naturally rich in vitamins and antioxidants from the apples. The nutritional content may vary depending on the specific brand of apple juice or cider used and any optional sweeteners added. It's a comforting drink suitable for those following the Anti-inflammatory Autoimmune Protocol (AIP), especially when made with unsweetened varieties of apple juice or cider.

Berry Kombucha

Ingredients:

1 gallon of prepared kombucha (homemade or store-bought)
1 cup mixed berries (such as raspberries, strawberries, blueberries)
Optional: Fresh herbs like mint or basil (for added flavor)
Optional: 1-2 tablespoons raw honey or maple syrup (omit for strict AIP)

Instructions:
1. Ensure your kombucha is already brewed and ready. If using store-bought, choose a plain, unflavored variety.
2. In a large glass jar or container, combine the mixed berries and optional herbs.
3. Pour the prepared kombucha over the berries, covering them completely.
4. If desired, stir in raw honey or maple syrup to sweeten (optional, omit for strict AIP).
5. Close the jar or container with a lid or cover it with a clean cloth secured with a rubber band.
6. Let the kombucha sit at room temperature for 2-3 days to allow the flavors to infuse. Taste occasionally to check the flavor intensity.
7. Once the desired flavor is achieved, strain the kombucha through a fine mesh sieve to remove the berries and herbs.
8. Transfer the berry kombucha into clean bottles with tight-sealing lids for storage.
9. Refrigerate the bottles to halt fermentation and chill before serving.

Tips/Notes:
Use organic berries whenever possible to avoid pesticides.
Adjust the sweetness and flavor intensity by varying the amount of berries and steeping time.
Kombucha is a fermented beverage with potential probiotic benefits. Ensure your brewing process is clean and sanitary.

Experiment with different berry combinations and herbs to create unique flavors.

Nutritional Information:
Kombucha is known for its probiotic content and potential health benefits, although specific nutritional values can vary based on fermentation time, ingredients, and brewing methods. This berry kombucha is a refreshing and probiotic-rich beverage option suitable for those following the Anti-inflammatory Autoimmune Protocol (AIP) when made with compliant ingredients.

VIII

7-Day Anti-Inflammatory protocol

Meal Plan

Creating a 7-day Anti-Inflammatory Protocol (AIP) meal plan focuses on nourishing the body with nutrient-dense foods while eliminating potential triggers for inflammation. Here's a guide to structuring such a meal plan:

Day 1:
Breakfast: AIP Breakfast Smoothie with mixed berries and coconut milk.
Lunch: Herb Roasted Chicken with a side of roasted vegetables.
Dinner: Grilled Salmon with steamed broccoli and a side salad dressed with olive oil and lemon.

Day 2:
Breakfast: Sweet Potato and Apple Hash topped with avocado.
Lunch: Turkey and Vegetable Soup.
Dinner: Baked Cod with Cauliflower "Rice" Stir Fry.

Day 3:
Breakfast: AIP Granola with Coconut Yogurt and fresh berries.
Lunch: Chicken Salad with mixed greens, cucumber, and AIP-friendly dressing.
Dinner: Beef Stir Fry with Zucchini Noodles.

Day 4:
Breakfast: Coconut Milk Chia Pudding topped with sliced kiwi.
Lunch: Butternut Squash Soup with a side of mixed greens.
Dinner: Herb-Infused Olive Oil Drizzled over Roasted Chicken Thighs and roasted root vegetables.

Day 5:
Breakfast: Plantain and Avocado Toast with a side of fresh fruit.
Lunch: AIP Chicken Tenders with a side of steamed broccoli.
Dinner: Stuffed Acorn Squash with Ground Turkey and Spinach.

Day 6:
Breakfast: Carrot and Zucchini Muffins with herbal tea.
Lunch: Cauliflower "Rice" with Pesto and Grilled Chicken.
Dinner: Roasted Vegetable Medley with baked fish.

Day 7:
Breakfast: Berry Chia Pudding with mixed nuts.
Lunch: AIP-Friendly Ketchup with Baked Sweet Potato Fries.
Dinner: Coconut Milk Chicken Curry with Cauliflower Rice.

This meal plan prioritizes fresh vegetables, lean proteins, healthy fats, and excludes grains, dairy, processed foods, and added sugars, aiming to support a balanced and anti-inflammatory diet. Adjust portions and ingredients to suit individual dietary needs and preferences while maintaining compliance with the AIP guidelines.

30-Day Challenge

A 30-day challenge focused on the Anti-Inflammatory Protocol (AIP) can be a transformative experience, designed to reset the body and reduce inflammation. Here's how to approach and benefit from a 30-day AIP challenge:

Setting Up Your 30-Day AIP Challenge

Preparation:
Begin by educating yourself about the AIP guidelines. This diet eliminates potential inflammatory foods such as grains, dairy, legumes, processed sugars, and nightshade vegetables while emphasizing nutrient-dense whole foods.

Meal Planning:
Create a comprehensive meal plan for the entire month, ensuring it includes a variety of AIP-compliant foods such as lean proteins (like poultry and fish), non-nightshade vegetables (such as sweet potatoes and leafy greens), healthy fats (like avocado and coconut oil), and fruits (except for high-sugar varieties).

Stocking Up:
Clear your pantry of non-compliant items and stock up on AIP-friendly staples like coconut milk, bone broth, herbal teas, and

fresh produce. Having these essentials on hand will simplify meal preparation and help you stay on track.

Benefits of a 30-Day AIP Challenge

Reduced Inflammation:
By eliminating potentially inflammatory foods, the AIP diet aims to reduce inflammation throughout the body. Many participants report improvements in joint pain, digestive issues, and overall well-being.

Improved Digestion:
The emphasis on whole foods and gut-friendly ingredients like bone broth and fermented foods supports digestive health and may alleviate symptoms such as bloating and gas.

Enhanced Energy Levels:
AIP encourages nutrient-dense meals that stabilize blood sugar levels and provide sustained energy throughout the day, reducing the highs and lows associated with processed foods.

Discovering Food Sensitivities:
Following a strict AIP protocol can help identify specific food sensitivities or triggers that may contribute to inflammation or digestive discomfort, allowing for personalized adjustments to optimize health.

Embracing Culinary Creativity:
The challenge encourages creativity in the kitchen, experimenting with new recipes and flavors that align with AIP principles. This can lead to a deeper appreciation for wholesome, nourishing meals.

Tips for Success

Stay Consistent: Commit fully to the 30-day challenge to experience the full benefits of the AIP diet.
Seek Support: Connect with online communities, support groups, or a healthcare professional knowledgeable about AIP for guidance and encouragement.
Monitor Progress: Keep a journal to track changes in symptoms, energy levels, and overall well-being throughout the challenge.
Plan Ahead: Prepare meals in advance and pack snacks to avoid temptation when dining out or during busy days.

Embarking on a 30-day AIP challenge can be a powerful step towards understanding your body's response to food and promoting long-term health and wellness through dietary choices.

Conversion Charts

Liquid Measurements

1 teaspoon (tsp) = 5 milliliters (ml)
1 tablespoon (Tbsp) = 15 milliliters (ml)
1 fluid ounce (fl oz) = 30 milliliters (ml)
1 cup = 240 milliliters (ml)
1 pint (pt) = 480 milliliters (ml) = 2 cups
1 quart (qt) = 960 milliliters (ml) = 4 cups
1 gallon (gal) = 3.8 liters (l) = 16 cups

Dry Measurements

1 teaspoon (tsp) = 5 grams (g)

1 tablespoon (Tbsp) = 15 grams (g)
1 ounce (oz) = 28 grams (g)
1 cup = 240 grams (g)
1 pound (lb) = 454 grams (g)
1 kilogram (kg) = 2.2 pounds (lbs)

Oven Temperature
250°F = 120°C = Gas Mark 1/2
275°F = 140°C = Gas Mark 1
300°F = 150°C = Gas Mark 2
325°F = 160°C = Gas Mark 3
350°F = 180°C = Gas Mark 4
375°F = 190°C = Gas Mark 5
400°F = 200°C = Gas Mark 6
425°F = 220°C = Gas Mark 7
450°F = 230°C = Gas Mark 8

Cups to Grams (Flour)
1 cup all-purpose flour = 120 grams
1 cup whole wheat flour = 130 grams
1 cup cake flour = 110 grams
1 cup bread flour = 125 grams

Common Ingredient Substitutions
1 cup buttermilk = 1 cup milk + 1 tablespoon vinegar or lemon juice
1 cup sour cream = 1 cup plain yogurt
1 cup sugar = 1 cup honey (reduce liquid in recipe by 1/4 cup)
1 cup butter = 1 cup margarine or 1 cup shortening

These conversion charts will help in adapting to the recipes of your preferred measurement systems and make substitutions when necessary. Adjust the details based on the specific needs and preferences of your choice and recipes.

Made in United States
Troutdale, OR
11/02/2024

24368313R00091